Breathe Easy:
mindful breathing made simple

by Martha DeSante DC, CYT

Cover and Image Design by: Michael Nelson

Photography by: Jessica Miller (three photos contributed by Paul DeSante)

Illustration by: Martha DeSante

Bonus Printable Breathe Art by: Gina Sekelsky of Lettergirl Studio

Wardrobe by: PrAna

I would like to thank many people for their help in making this book possible, including my family, all of my teachers, Jessica Miller, Gina Sekelsky, and especially Michael Nelson. Thank you all so much for sharing your gifts with me so that I can more beautifully convey this information. Michael, thank you for always sticking with me, encouraging me, and inspiring me to bring my dreams into being.

A big thank you goes out to Paul DeSante. Thank you for always supporting me, believing in me and loving me – in the creation of <u>Breathe Easy</u>, in my practice and in life. Thank you for appreciating my obsession with how the body is put together and how it works, or "bones and yoga" as you like to say. It is with your loving kindness that I am able to live my purpose. You inspire so much love and deep gratitude in my heart. Thank you!

I would also like to thank you, dear reader, for taking the time to make yourself a priority! Thank you for loving you and for continuing to learn and grow. I know your breath practice will enrich your life and the lives of those around you. Just keep showing up to the practice every day and the rest will take care of itself.

I dedicate this book to the memory of the first person who taught me about the importance of breath; my mother Freda June Tarbell.

Please enjoy this introduction to mindful breathing! As always, use caution when performing any new physical activity. If something doesn't feel right, please stop practicing that particular exercise until you can get clarification on what changes you can make to safely continue. Not every activity is a good fit for every person all of the time, so be sure to follow up if you are receiving warning signs from your body (pain, anxiety, etc.). Sometimes something as small as a simple modification can shift an exercise from being inappropriate for an individual to being safe and effective, so be sure to consult a knowledgeable practitioner if you have questions.

This information is designed to enhance your relationship with your own body. By better knowing your own body and taking care of it, this will enhance your relationship with your health care providers. The information in this book is not meant to take the place of that relationship. If you have a particular health concern, please seek treatment from a qualified health care provider! If you have any questions about your ability to safely engage in this (or any) breath or movement program, please get the okay from your doctor first. Be safe and have fun!

Table of Contents

Hello! My name is Martha DeSante and I am so excited to offer you this transformational breath work practice! The following information is a combination of knowledge and techniques drawn from my experience singing in professional choirs, training in yoga and Pilates instruction and education and practice as a Doctor of Chiropractic. This program combines diverse techniques and ideas to create the foundation for your own intentional breathing practice.

I want to congratulate you for choosing loving self-care in the form of this intentional breathing practice. For best results, I recommend that you PRACTICE EVERY DAY. You can devote as much or as little time as you feel is appropriate... just remember that this is one of those opportunities where you get out of the practice what you put into it.

I will be using the terms "mindful breathing" and "intentional breathing" interchangeably. All mindful or intentional breathing means is that we will be paying attention to our breath. It really is as simple as that. Intentional breathing is a great practice for many reasons. Intentional breathing is something that you can practice anywhere, and you don't need any fancy or expensive equipment. You can begin at any age or fitness level to improve your well being right now. Your breath practice will enhance and support you in whatever other activities you're already doing.

Intentional breathing is also a simple tool with profound effects that can help us get out of the swift current of thoughts flowing through our head and into a grounded experience of life in our body. If you have always wanted to try meditation and weren't sure where or how to start, today is your day! Meditation can be quite simple and approachable. It doesn't have to be something that feels complicated or intimidating. All it takes to begin a meditative breathing practice is applying your loving dedication and shining the brilliant light of your awareness on something that we take for granted on a daily basis... our breath!

I wish you love and luck as you begin your breathing adventure! Please explore the Bonus! pages to print the companion Breathe Easy journal now if you would like to use that as an additional resource.

Chapter One
What Does Breathing Do for Me?

With every activity that requires time and dedication, most people have one question... What's in it for me? We'll touch on the basics of what breathing does for our bodies now and get into more detail in a little bit.

Breathing brings fresh oxygen into the body and gets carbon dioxide out of the body. When we breathe in, oxygen comes into our lungs and it is transferred to our blood, which then carries the oxygen to all of our cells and tissues. The blood picks up carbon dioxide and other waste products from our cells and carries it back to our lungs, where it is released as we exhale. In this way, efficient breathing keeps our cells and tissues fresh and energized. Breathing well also helps to keep our thinking clear because the brain, even more than other organs, really needs a steady supply of oxygen to do its job well.

We could think of our breath as the most important element in maintaining our health. If we think about the things that we typically associate with a healthy lifestyle, such as food, water, and sleep, none can compare in the role of maintaining our health and even sustaining our life. Another way to think about this is that we can go for quite a while without food and still survive - maybe a few weeks. We can go slightly less long without sleep and water - maybe a few days - and still recover. We can't survive more than a few minutes without breathing.

If you are someone who wants to know more about how breathing can improve your life and why you would want to develop a mindful breathing practice, feel free to jump ahead to read Chapters 14 and 15 before you continue. If you are ready to start connecting with your breath in a physical, experiential way right now, please continue on to Chapter 2!

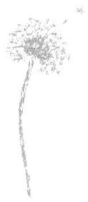

You can make the choice to be either sitting or standing for these exercises. In whatever position you have chosen, feel your feet flat on the floor, a comfortable distance apart.

If you are sitting, feel your sitting bones (those bony points at the base of your butt) press downward gently into your chair. Sit with your back upright and away from the back of your chair if you can.

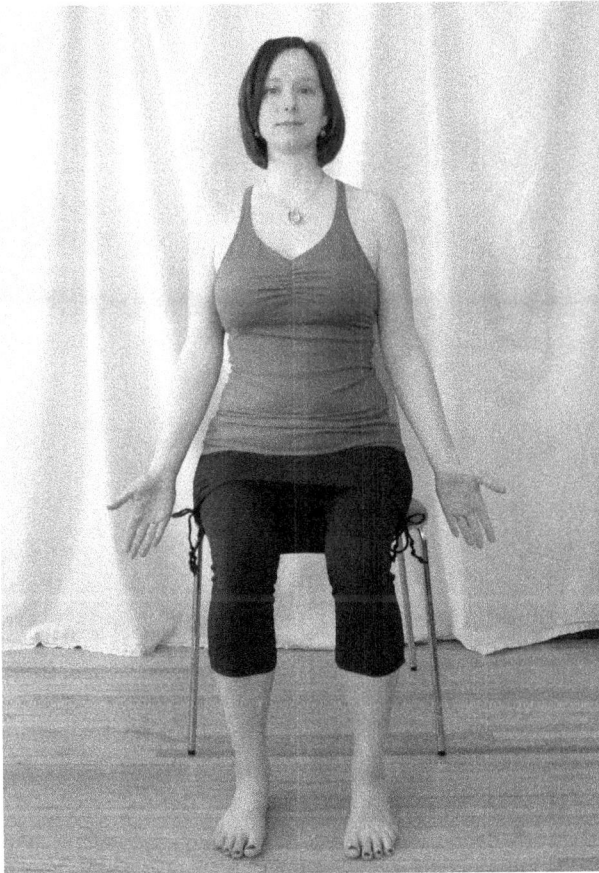

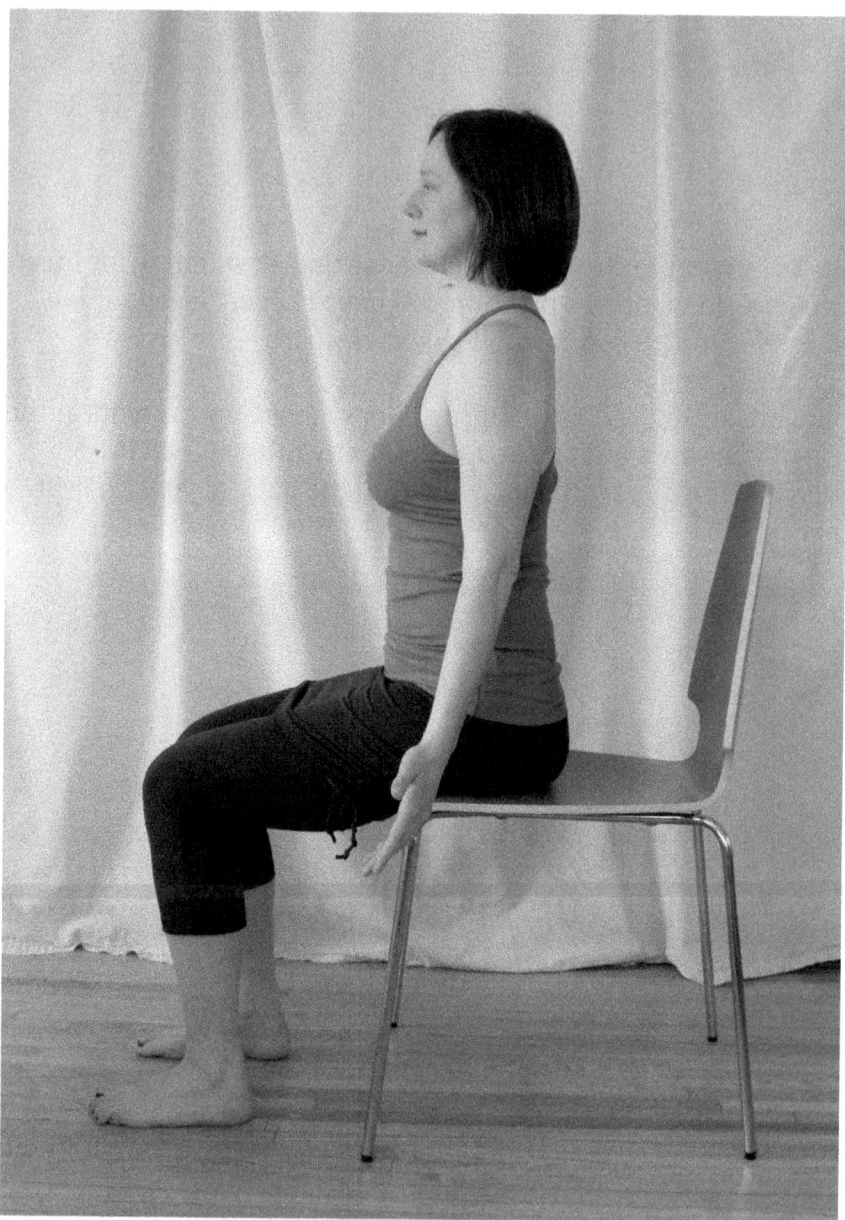

If you are standing, maintain that grounded connection with your feet. Allow your weight to shift back toward your heels slightly so that you can lift and wiggle your toes. Let your knees stay straight yet soft. If you have a tendency toward "locking out" the knee joints, keep a little micro-bend in your knees.

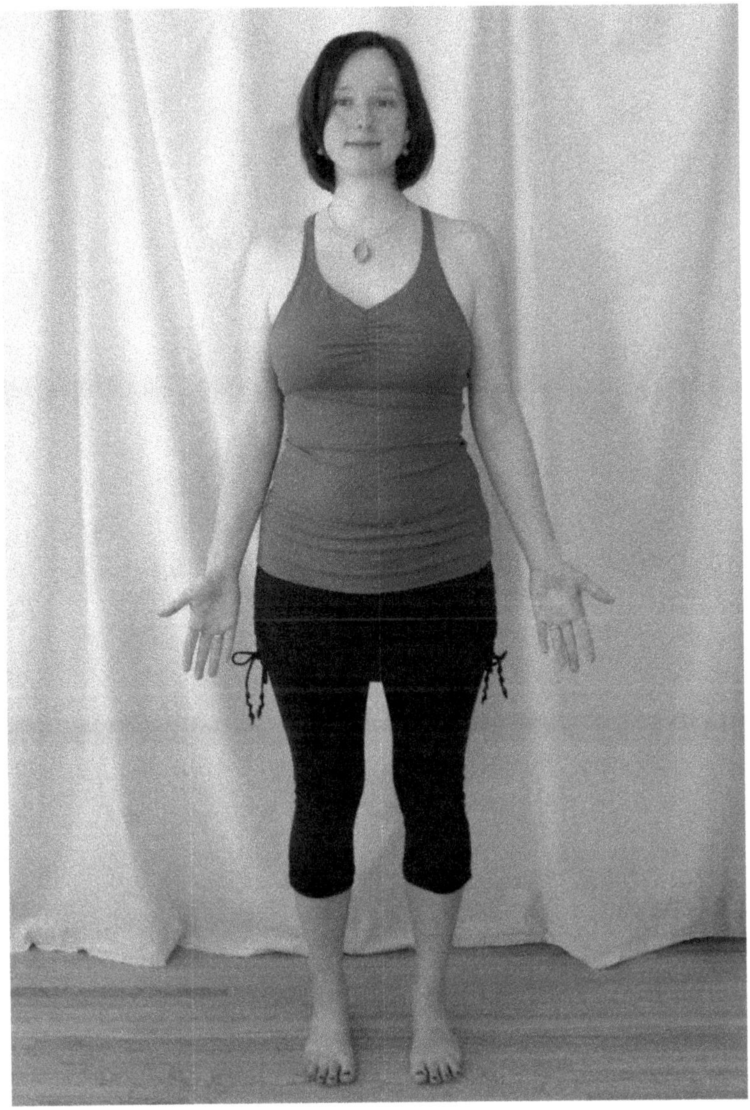

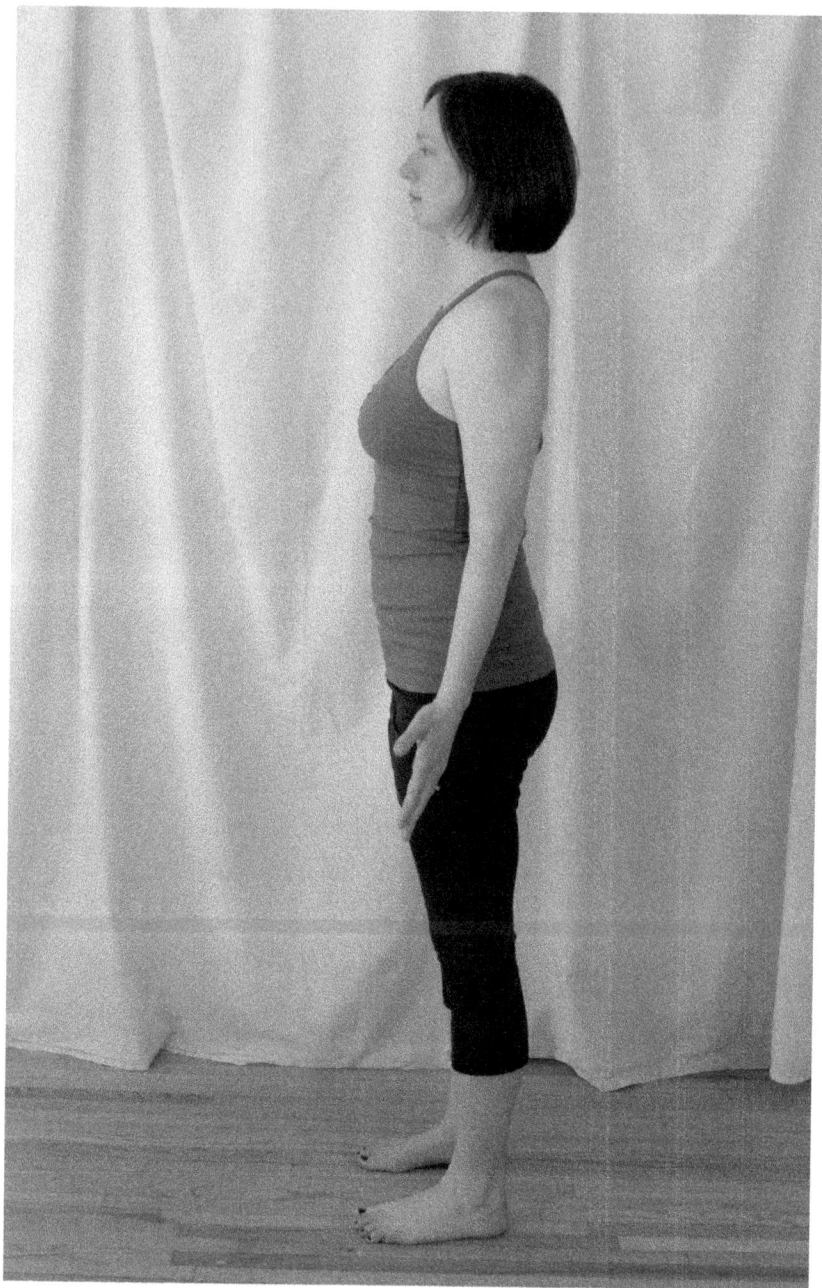

Allow your spine and the crown of your head to lengthen upward toward the sky from this firm foundation. Take a moment to feel your breath right now without changing anything.

Simply by bringing your awareness to your breath you may notice that it is already beginning to change. If your breath becomes more full and deep, make a mental note that this is what your body is naturally calling for when you make the time and space to listen to it.

Now we are going to try an experiment... there is no right or wrong here and no judgment. This is all about just noticing what is. In this experiment, you are a scientist objectively observing your breath.

Become aware of the rate of your breath, whether it feels fast or slow.

Notice the depth of your breath, whether it feels shallow or deep.

Check in with the quality of your breath, noticing whether it is flowing smoothly or has rough edges.

Notice if there is any sound associated with your breath.

Are there are any emotions or feelings associated with this experience of your breath?

Allow yourself to suspend any judgment about whether the way you are breathing is "good" or "bad" and let your self be fully present with what is.

Notice where you feel your breath moving in your body.

Take 3 more breaths like this.

Maintain this connection to your breath as we move forward. If you would like to close your eyes and focus on your breath, feel free to do so now for several breaths. When you feel ready, gently blink your eyes open.

Journal Opportunity #1

What are your initial impressions? Write down any
observations that feel important to you about this first
awareness based experience with your breath in your
Breathe Easy journal now.

What are your initial impressions? Write down any observations
that feel important to you about this first awareness based
experience with your breath in your Breathe Easy journal now.

Chapter Three

A Note of Caution

At this point, I want to mention a brief note of caution. While we have all been breathing every day since birth, working with the breath in ways we aren't used to may make some people feel dizzy or light headed. If at any time you feel dizzy or light headed, please sit or lie down and return to your own quiet breathing pattern until this sensation passes. Over time and with practice, your body will get used to a more full breath pattern.

This program is designed to provide you with the opportunity to enjoy the benefits of mindful breathing while utilizing very gentle and safe techniques. There may be specific individuals who would benefit from a slightly modified approach due to their unique history or conditions.

If you have any medical conditions, specifically conditions affecting your lung or heart function, please talk with your doctor before beginning this or any breathing program to determine if any modifications should be made for you.

Chapter Four

Tips For Success – Breath Check-in
Where's the Breath?

As you go thru the program for the first time, keep in mind that there is a lot of information presented. Be kind and patient with yourself, especially if intentional breathing is new to you. As your breathing practice grows and develops, you can begin to unpack different layers that you may not have understood in the beginning. If you feel like you don't understand all the information at first, that's okay! You will learn and benefit more from repeated reading and practice.

If it's possible when and where you are practicing, take off any tight fitting clothing - especially belts, bras or pants with tight waistbands. These things can hinder the natural movement of the ribs and the belly. Obviously there will be some situations where this isn't possible, so do the best you can with the opportunity you have. You may be surprised to find that over time you begin to choose more "breathing friendly" clothing that doesn't restrict your movement.

Good riddance to bad rubbish!

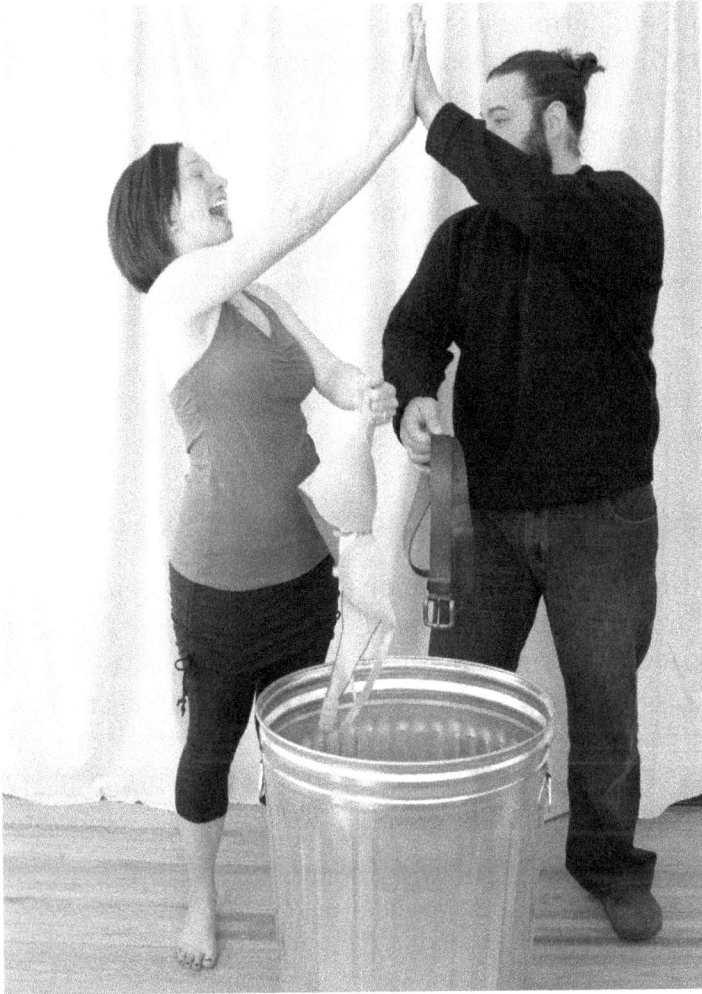

Maybe this will be our holiday card this year?
"Have a relaxing holiday letting it all hang out!"

Another way you can ensure your success is by letting go of the need to do things "right". Our minds can quickly jump in and criticize our efforts. This distracts us and takes the fun out of our experience. Don't let your mind hijack this experience and fill you with worry about if what you're doing is "right" or "wrong". Instead, learn to enjoy exploring! Let yourself be objectively curious to learn more about yourself and your breath. Be that scientist... this is all just an experiment after all.

Give yourself permission to take in as much information as feels good to you each time you engage with this material. There may come a point where it feels like there is no more room in your brain for anything else. If that happens, let go of any effort or grasping for information and just feel your breath. Even though it may not seem like it, your gorgeous brain is doing something with that information. Behind the scenes, your brain is laying the foundation for you to gain an even deeper understanding of this material when you encounter it again in the future.

Let yourself trust the process and realize that you will get exactly what you need from your practice today.

CHECK BACK IN

So now that you've been reading for a while, let's check back in with your breath. Did that feel like a sneaky trick? To get you reading and thinking about other things, then ask "where's the breath?" This is why it is important to devote at least a few minutes each day to practicing full breathing, so full breathing becomes something that we are used to. When breathing fully becomes a practiced skill, we don't always have to think about it to be able to breathe well.

Journal Opportunity #2

Did you maintain connection with your breath easily while continuing to read? Did your breathing revert to a different pattern? Write down any observations that feel important to you about this second awareness based experience with your breath in your Breathe Easy journal now.

Did you maintain connection with your breath easily while continuing to read? Did your breathing revert to a different pattern? Write down any observations that feel important to you about this second awareness based experience with your breath in your Breathe Easy journal now.

Take a moment and reconnect with your strong foundation. Feel your feet connected to the earth. If you are sitting, feel your sitting bones connected with the seat of your chair below.

Let your spine lengthen up from this strong base, sitting – or standing - tall with the crown of your head reaching up to the sky. Feel your shoulders shrug up to your ears, then gently slide down your back and remain relaxed there.

Again notice how fast or slow your breath feels right now.

Become aware of how shallow or deep your breath feels.

Check in with how smooth or jagged your breath feels.

Notice any sounds or emotions that accompany your breath.

Gradually invite your breath to become more full and deep.

Notice where you feel your breath moving in your body.

Keep this full breath pattern going for several more breaths. If it helps you to focus on your breath, you may close your eyes. When you feel ready, gently blink your eyes open.

WHERE ARE YOU FEELING YOUR BREATH MOVING IN YOUR BODY?

My big question for you now is this... Where did you feel your breath moving in your body? If you aren't sure, allow your eyes to close and take five full breaths while being open to feeling the sensation of the breath moving through the body. If you still aren't sure after trying the five breaths, that's okay too.

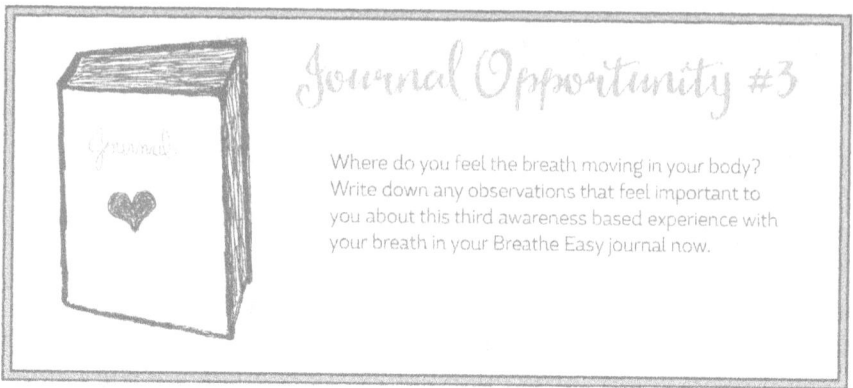

Where do you feel the breath moving in your body? Write down any observations that feel important to you about this third awareness based experience with your breath in your Breathe Easy journal now.

Many of us only feel movement of the breath in the area of the upper chest and on the front of the body when we first start our breathing practice. This is called chest breathing and it is a very common pattern. It's also really inefficient and can cause a lot of tension in the neck and upper shoulders. If you know you hold tension in this area of your body, it is very likely that you are doing a lot of chest breathing. Chest breathing can contribute to neck and upper shoulder tension and discomfort as the accessory (or helper) muscles used in breathing that are located in the neck have to work harder when we aren't letting our diaphragm move fully.

Shallow breathing patterns like chest breathing could be described as "maintenance breathing"... really just enough to keep us alive and going. Maintenance breath isn't wrong or bad, it's absolutely vital. Imagine how exhausting it would be if you had to think about every breath. Many of us are very fortunate and have been breathing since birth without having to think about it at all. Our bodies are so incredibly cool! Without having to do anything, we breathe, our hearts beat, and our food is turned into energy we can use to run our body.

Take a moment to feel deep gratitude for your body and all of the amazing things that it allows you to do every day.

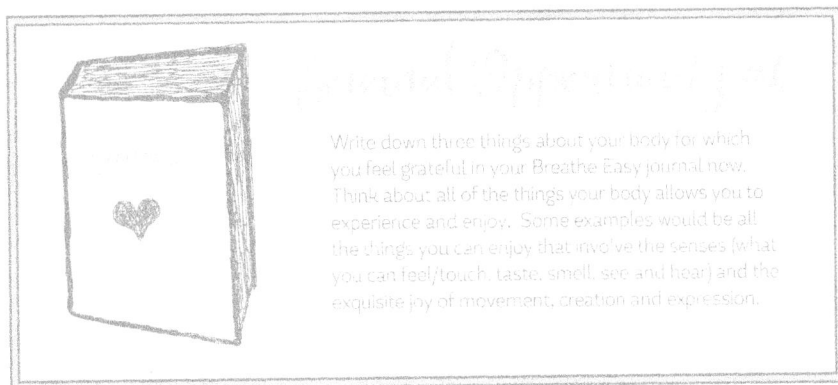

Write down three things about your body for which you feel grateful in your Breathe Easy journal now. Think about all of the things your body allows you to experience and enjoy. Some examples would be all the things you can enjoy that involve the senses (what you can feel/touch, taste, smell, see and hear) and the exquisite joy of movement, creation and expression.

Let's return to our breath movement check-in experience. Where did you feel the air entering and leaving your body? When you were just practicing this last awareness exercise, were you breathing through your nose or your mouth? Which way do you usually breathe? If you were breathing through your nose, did it feel difficult or relatively easy? If you are congested or unable to breathe through your nose without stress or strain, please breathe through your mouth.

Ideally, we breathe through the nose as often as we are able. Breathing through the nose filters, warms and humidifies the air before it comes into our lungs. Breathing through the nose also produces nitric oxide, which kills bacteria and increases oxygen-carrying ability in the body, helping you to get more oxygen to your blood and tissues with each breath.

There are many reasons why it may feel challenging to breathe through your nose. As a reformed mouth breather, I am personally familiar with many of these obstacles to breathing through the nose. Allergies, a deviated septum, habitual mouth breathing due to tongue tie/orofacial abnormalities or a respiratory illness can all cause mouth breathing. Breathing through the mouth is associated with many undesirable health outcomes, so it is preferable to breathe through your nose as often as you are able.

Something that may make breathing through your nose easier is evaluating the position of your tongue in your mouth. Take a moment to notice where your tongue rests in your mouth right now as you breathe through your nose with your mouth closed. Ideally the tongue rests at the roof of the mouth with the top surface of the tongue gently contacting the palate. In my own personal experience, I have noticed that breathing with the tongue at the roof of the mouth rather than resting on the floor of the mouth, makes breathing through my nose much easier. It may take time to retrain your tongue to rest at the roof of your mouth if you have previously held it in a resting position at the floor of the mouth. It is also entirely possible to learn this new position as long as the tongue has the required strength and mobility. If you find that you can't comfortably bring your tongue to rest on the roof of your mouth, you may benefit from a consult with a dentist who evaluates for the presence of tongue tie (there are many grades, so a subtle tongue tie may not be noticeable to an untrained eye) as well as an orofacial myofunctional therapist.

Another interesting element to consider when checking in with what's happening inside the mouth is the condition of the jaw and teeth. If you bring your awareness to your jaw how does it feel right now? Is it relatively relaxed, is it tightly clenched, or is it somewhere in between? Allow your teeth to part slightly while your lips remain closed. Feel the muscles of the jaw release. Gently bring the teeth back together. Allow yourself to take five full breaths right now with the top surface of the tongue gently resting against the roof of the mouth, the teeth gently touching, the jaw relaxed and the lips closed. Take a moment to check in with how that feels.

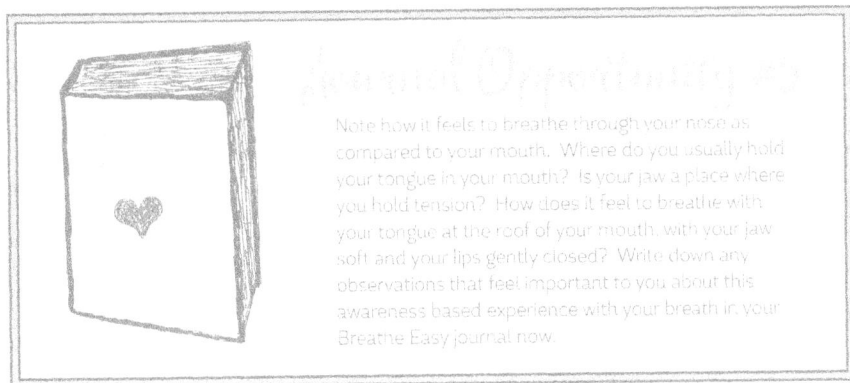

Note how it feels to breathe through your nose as compared to your mouth. Where do you usually hold your tongue in your mouth? Is your jaw a place where you hold tension? How does it feel to breathe with your tongue at the roof of your mouth, with your jaw soft and your lips gently closed? Write down any observations that feel important to you about this awareness based experience with your breath in your Breathe Easy journal now.

Something else to consider when breathing fully, especially through the nose, is our comfort with breaking the sound barrier. In social or work situations have you ever noticed that you were breathing in a very shallow and quiet fashion in order to not make any noise? Most people feel some amount of discomfort when making sounds that may draw the attention of other people around them. If you have a deviated septum or nasal congestion, the added resistance as air passes through your nose may cause your breath to be more audible. Once we become aware of any discomfort around making sounds when we breathe deeply, we can begin to work through that discomfort and choose to breathe in a way that improves our health and vitality… even if that means other people may hear us.

A different way to think about this is that by breathing well you are taking good care of yourself and setting a healthy example for other people in your life. Many of us have had the experience of hearing someone taking a full breath and then becoming aware of our own breathing, often taking a deeper breath or two after noticing that subconscious breathing prompt. When other people hear you breathing, you are reminding them of how good it feels to take a deep breath and encouraging them to check in with their own breathing without saying a word.

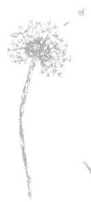

Since we now know that chest breathing isn't the best option for getting oxygen into our bodies, let's talk about how we can begin to make use of more of our lung space rather than just that front, top portion. The first step in being able to use all of our lung space is to become aware of where it is. One way to think about all the lung space you have is that if there are ribs around it, there is lung tissue in it! The rib cage wraps from the back of the body at the spine, around the sides and joins together at the sternum – or breastbone – at the front of the body. There are some other organs protected by the rib cage, but the lungs do fill most of the space of the rib cage on ALL sides of the body. Imagine if we took full advantage of all of that lung space every time we took a breath in and out!

Some good inspiration for your breath practice is to watch a baby or a pet breathe. When we were born, we used to breathe with our whole body. Babies and animals still breathe this way. When we strip off all of our hang-ups and get out of our own way, the breath breathes us, rather than the other way around. This means that right now you aren't learning anything new... you are returning to your natural way of breathing by peeling off layers of cultural conditioning, stress and postural restriction. You are coming home to your breath.

There are many different breath techniques that you can use for different activities. I'm not suggesting that any one technique or exercise is better than another. I do think that there is a huge benefit to understanding the breath and being able to choose what breath pattern best supports you in whatever activity you are doing at the time.

When in doubt, allow yourself to return to a full, smooth, natural breath pattern. While it sounds like this should come "naturally" to all of us, unfortunately a full, natural breath pattern has been conditioned out of most of us through stress and cultural pressures. Let's start shedding those restrictive layers and talk about what that full, natural breath pattern looks like right now!

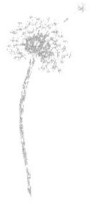

Chapter Six

Breathing Into the Front of the Body – Belly Love

We'll start with an awareness exercise where we focus on breathing on the front side of the body. Unless you are congested, let's breathe in and out through the nose. If you are having difficulty breathing through your nose, please feel free to breathe through your mouth. Allow the breath to flow freely and smoothly in and out, with no pause between inhale and exhale.

Connect with your foundation - feeling your feet on the floor, your seat grounding if you're sitting - then lengthen upward from that strong base.

When you take a breath in, visualize your breath traveling in and down through your nostrils, chest and abdomen, until it fills your pelvic bowl.

As you breathe out, visualize the breath traveling up and out through your abdomen and chest, then exiting through your nostrils.

When we breathe in, we allow our belly to gently soften and expand outward and downward.

When we breathe out, we gently draw our belly inward and upward to press out any stale air that may be lingering in the lower parts of our lungs.

While we breathe smoothly and fully this way, our neck and shoulders stay soft and relaxed.

Keep this full breath pattern coming while we talk about abdominal –or- belly breathing.

The reason that the belly moves as we inhale and exhale has to do with a very important muscle for breathing... our diaphragm! The diaphragm is a large, dome-shaped sheet of muscle that is located just beneath the ribcage. It's not only at the front side of the body, but runs all the way through the body from front to back and from side to side. The diaphragm separates the torso into the chest above and the abdomen below. It is also the main muscle used in a full healthy breathing pattern!

As we inhale, our diaphragm pulls downward, changing the pressure in the chest so that air is drawn into the lungs. As we exhale, the diaphragm draws back up to assist in pressing air out of the chest. When the diaphragm draws down as we breathe in, our abdominal organs have to go somewhere to let the diaphragm move fully – that is why the belly relaxes outward as we breathe in. As we exhale, the diaphragm draws back upward and our belly can draw in and up back toward the spine. In the following photos, my hands are placed about where the diaphragm is located to show this motion.

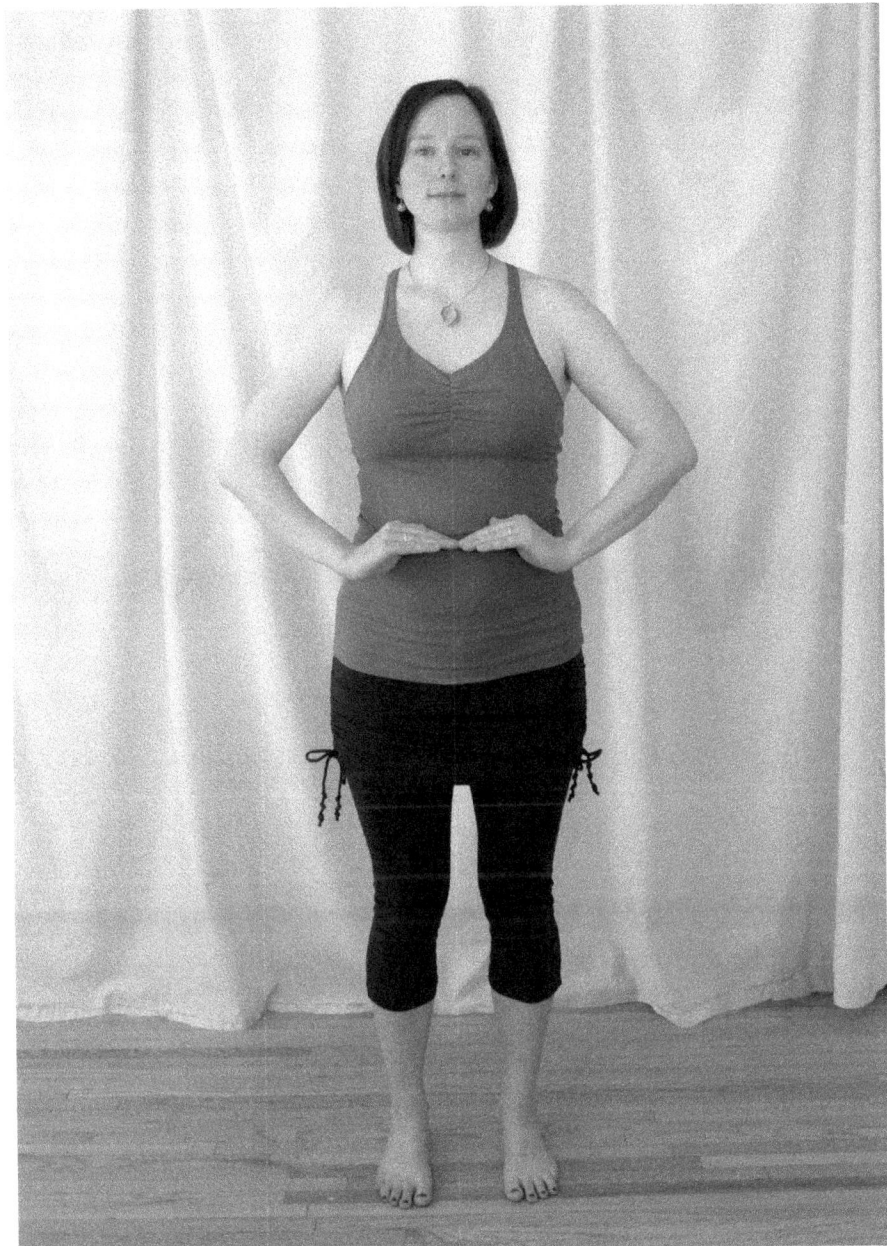

Inhale and the diaphragm pulls downward

Exhale and the diaphragm draws upward

When we don't allow our diaphragm to move fully because we are holding our belly in tight, this restriction can contribute to pain and dysfunction in several areas of the body. We touched on the way that chest breathing can lead to tension and pain in the neck and upper shoulders, due to the overuse of the accessory breathing muscles like the scalene and sternocleidomastoid muscles. These muscles are designed to be used to help us breathe when we are really physically active and our diaphragm needs a little bit of back up. We may also use those muscles when we are having difficulty breathing due to an illness or a condition like asthma. They are not intended to do the majority of our breathing work, and overuse of these muscles through chest breathing can lead to chronic neck and shoulder pain and tension.

Another area that suffers when we suck in our stomach and don't allow our diaphragm to move is the low back. There is a correlation established between chronic low back pain and abnormal breathing patterns. When the diaphragm and the belly aren't allowed to move freely, there is an increase in abdominal pressure as we inhale that can cause an increase in pressure on the spinal structures. This increase in pressure can exacerbate symptoms in people who are managing spinal disc injuries.

The health and function of our pelvic floor can be negatively impacted by always holding the belly tight, too. It is essential for the belly to relax outward and downward as we inhale to prevent excessive pressures from pushing upward into the chest cavity above the diaphragm, backward toward the spinal structures and downward into the pelvic floor. When we hold tension in our abdomen, we also usually hold tension in our pelvic floor. This combination of chronically held tension in the pelvic floor and the abnormal pressure exerted on the pelvic floor when the belly is held rigidly can contribute to pelvic floor dysfunction and urinary leaking.

BODY LOVE TIP

Embracing and loving our bellies can help us to breathe better. Sometimes, people develop a reverse breathing pattern, where they are "sucking it in" on the inhale and letting the belly drop on the exhale. Sometimes there really isn't much movement happening in the belly at all and the abdominal muscles are constantly kept in a guarded state of contraction. Neither of these options are natural or particularly effective breath patterns. They are developed through fear, cultural influence and the idea of "sucking in the gut".

This is where it becomes important to get comfortable with the idea of letting our belly soften. Many of us hold our belly in all the time to appear more slender and fit. While it is important to be able to contract our abdominal muscles quickly, strongly and effectively for many different activities, it is just as important to learn how to relax them.

Any patterns of chronic holding, contraction and shortening don't serve our bodies well. This contributes to maladaptive energetic holding patterns as well as to physical tightness and imbalances. A strong muscle isn't one that is always tightly clenched. A strong muscle is one that can alternate between a relaxed and contracted state in a responsive, coordinated way.

If you think about this same sort of chronic holding pattern with a muscle like your bicep, keeping the bicep constantly in a state of contraction really doesn't allow for any functional use of that muscle. You need to be able to have that full range from contracted to relaxed in order for that muscle to be functionally useful and effective.

I'm strong to the finish, 'cause I eat me spinach! It's hard to actually do anything with this arm when I'm flexing all the time...

Your arm isn't able to perform its full range of motion if the bicep muscle is constantly kept tightly contracted. This restricted range of motion severely limits the functional ability of your arm. The abdominal muscles also need to be able to move through their full range of motion to maintain full health and functionality.

Breathing fully and allowing the belly and the diaphragm to go through their full ranges of motion will gently massage the abdominal organs, allowing them to release waste products and draw in fresh oxygen from the blood. A supple belly, responsive, soft and strong, is what will serve us the best in our breath practice and in life.

When we are thinking about contracting the abdominal muscles, the action is a flattening and broadening of the belly on the exhale as the belly draws gently in and up. We are using the deep abdominal muscles (particularly the transversus abdominis) to help us perform a full and active exhale. When we exhale fully, we are clearing out as much stale air from the lungs as possible, making room for fresh oxygen rich air.

Let's try this diaphragmatic or belly breathing now.

Place your hands on your belly and as you inhale, feel your breath moving in and down to fill your hands. This motion is not pushing the belly outward, but rather allowing it to soften passively with your inhale.

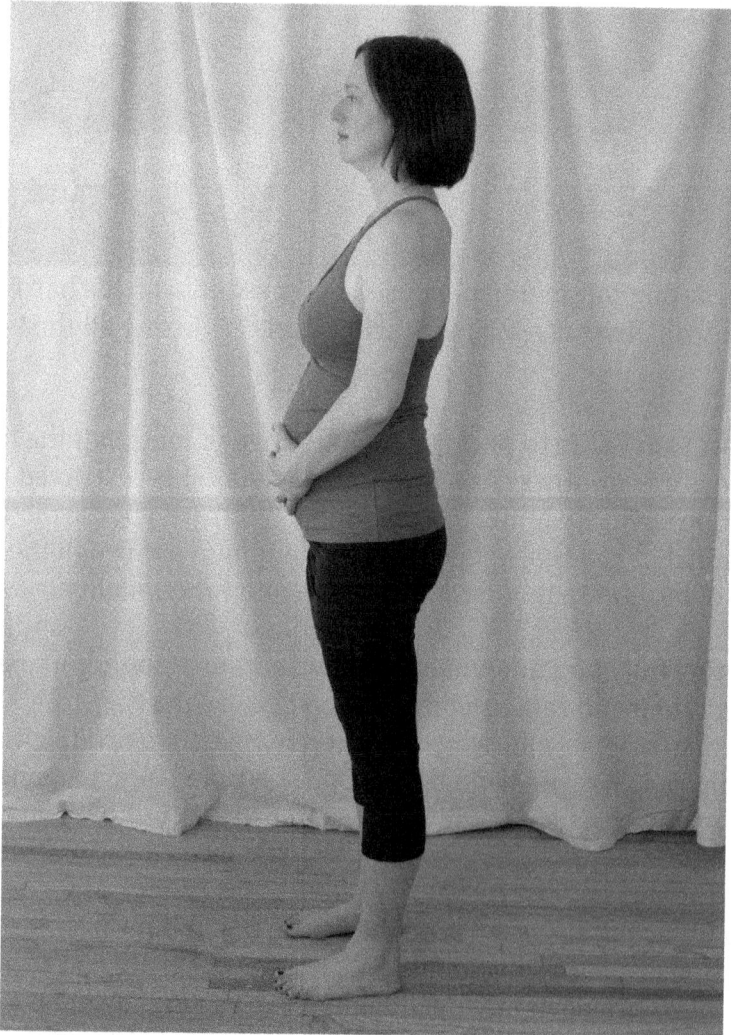

INHALE

As you breathe out, feel your belly draw in and up, toward your spine and away from your hands.

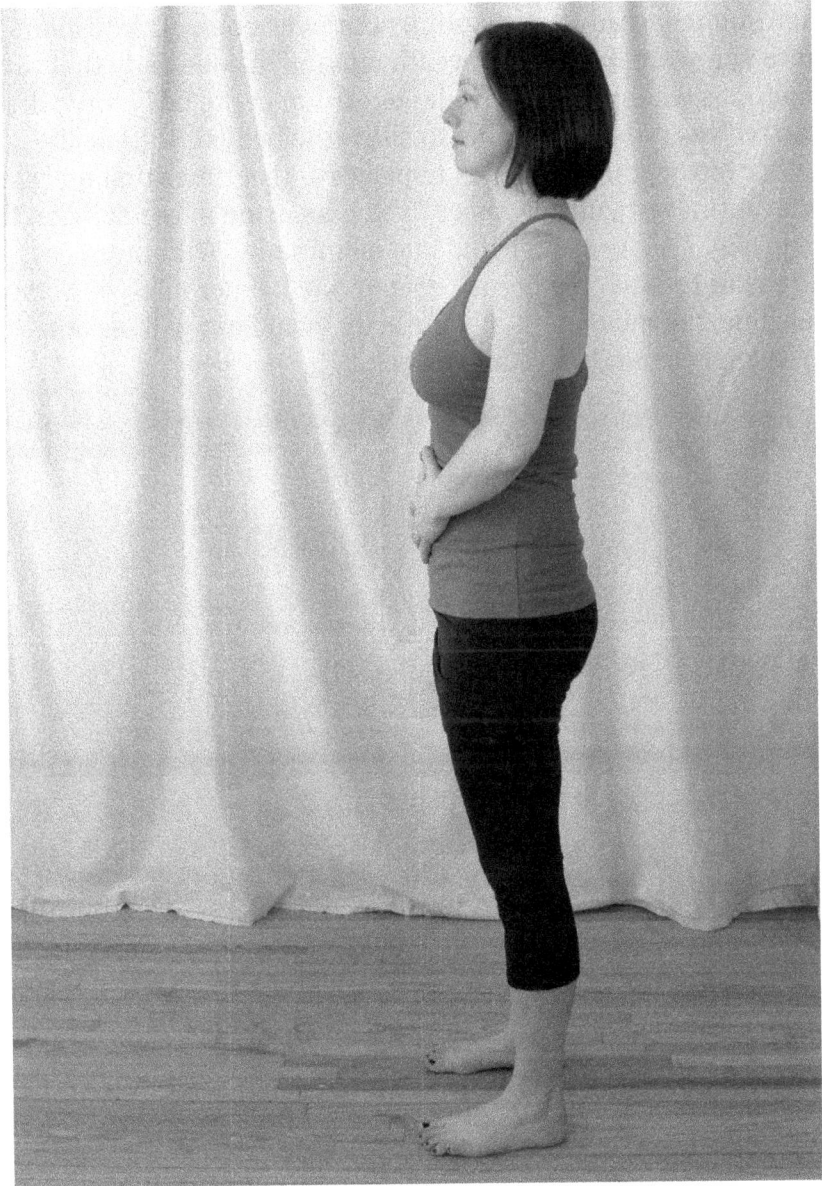

EXHALE

Allow yourself to take five more full breaths like that. You may close your eyes and focus on your breath and sensations if that is helpful to you.

When you feel ready, gently blink your eyes open. Think about where you were feeling the breath moving in your body that time. Sometimes when people have held tension in the belly for years, it can feel scary or impossible to allow the belly to soften. Practice letting the belly relax in places and at times that feel safe and eventually it will get easier. The expansion of the belly on the inhale may also feel rough and jagged initially. With practice it gets easier to draw the breath deeper and deeper into your body. Over time, the movement of your belly in and out will become increasingly smooth, free and easy.

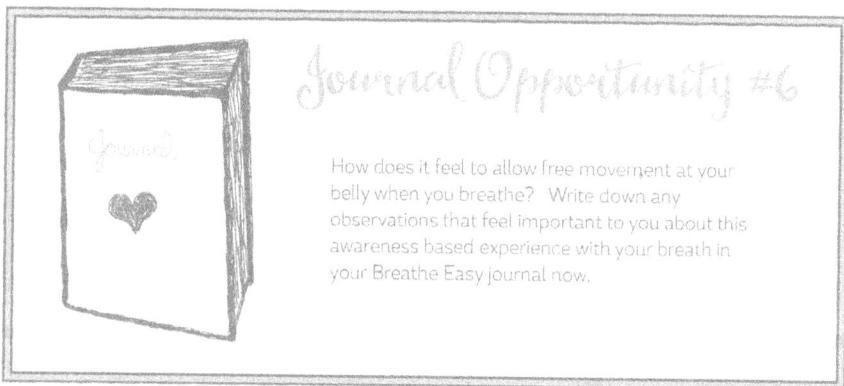

Journal Opportunity #6

How does it feel to allow free movement at your belly when you breathe? Write down any observations that feel important to you about this awareness based experience with your breath in your Breathe Easy journal now.

How does it feel to allow free movement at your belly when you breathe? Write down any observations that feel important to you about this awareness based experience with your breath in your Breathe Easy journal now.

BLOW OUT THE CANDLE

Another way to connect with the diaphragm and the TA is to use an exercise called "blow out the candle". This type of breath is practiced with an inhale through the nose and a strong, quick exhale out the mouth through pursed lips, just as if you were blowing out a candle. When practicing this technique, let your shoulders and neck stay relaxed. It can be helpful to breathe like this during strenuous activity when you want to blow off accumulating carbon dioxide without the added resistance of breathing out through your nose.

Lets try 5 breaths like that right now.

Notice what's happening at your belly when you breathe like this. Your belly should soften as you breathe in, and draw in as you blow the air out.

Lets try 5 more breaths that way, focusing on the movement at the belly.

Now take three full smooth breaths and check in with how you feel after that experience.

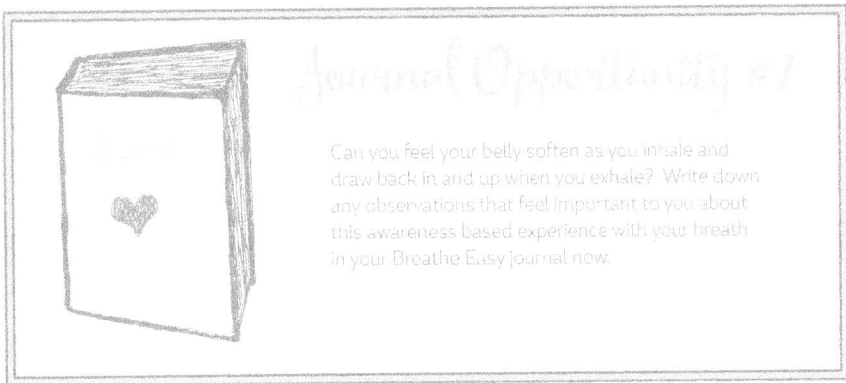

Can you feel your belly soften as you inhale and draw back in and up when you exhale? Write down any observations that feel important to you about this awareness based experience with your breath in your Breathe Easy journal now.

If you are still having difficulty with allowing the belly to move with the breath, if you are someone breathing with a reverse pattern, or if you are looking for a way to strengthen your diaphragm, here is another exercise to try. This is something we would do to strengthen our diaphragms when I sang in a children's church choir. In that setting, we always used hymnals – though you could use any sort of books, a small yoga sandbag, a bag of rice - really anything that provides gentle weight on the abdomen and does not cause you any discomfort. Please do not practice this technique if you have had recent abdominal surgery, if you are pregnant, or if it causes you any pain or anxiety. Gather whatever object you plan to use as your gentle weight to place on your belly. Lie down on your back with your knees bent and your feet on the floor about hip distance apart. Place one or both hands on your abdomen and notice as your belly gently rises and falls with the breath. When you feel ready, gently place your item on your belly, near the base of the ribcage. As you inhale, the object on your belly will raise upward. As you exhale, the object on your belly will lower back toward your spine. Spend some time breathing like this with the weighted object on the belly. When you feel ready, remove this item and set it off to the side. Connect with your breathing again and notice if anything has changed. This increased feedback may make it easier to feel the free movement at the belly and assist in retraining the habits of people who breathe in a reversed pattern.

Chapter Seven

Breathing Into the Basement
– Pelvic Floor...the Belly's BFF

Now it's time to take a moment to talk about the deep abdominal muscles best friends... the deep muscles of the pelvic floor! The muscles of the pelvic floor act as a muscular hammock that gives support to your body at the base of the pelvis. These muscles span from the pubic bones in the front to the tailbone in the back and side-to-side from one sitting bone to the other. They support our internal organs as well as helping us to stabilize our spine.

It's not uncommon to lose connection with these muscles in the same way you could lose touch with a friend if you don't communicate regularly. In the beginning, it may feel tricky to connect with the pelvic floor if you have not attempted to "talk" with your pelvic floor in a long time – or ever. If you have had any trauma to the tissues of the pelvic floor resulting from childbirth, surgery or injury, please be patient and kind with yourself. You may not feel your pelvic floor muscles moving as we work on this next component. If that is the case, don't worry. With practice eventually you will re-establish this connection. For now just stay open to the possibility of feeling connection and movement at the pelvic floor in the future.

The pelvic floor, like the belly, is also a common area where we may hold tension without being aware of it. If you encounter resistance to the movement of the breath and to sensation in the pelvic floor, don't be discouraged. Invite your breath to begin to move gently into this area. Take your time and be compassionate with yourself. Honor any resistance or emotion that accompanies this work.

If you have experienced sexual trauma, proceed with gentle awareness. If working with increased breath and awareness in the lower abdomen and pelvic floor begins to bring up emotions, continue breathing, honor these feelings and proceed at your own pace. The body can hold experiences in its tissues, and it is possible that working with the body and breath can begin to draw out stored information about such experiences. Using the breath and awareness to release and move through these experiences can be highly beneficial. Please reach out for all of the help and support you need, whether it be from friends, family members or supportive professionals like psychotherapists, so that you can move into a greater space of integration and healing through this experience.

The pelvic floor naturally moves in a manner similar to the respiratory diaphragm that we talked about before. As we inhale, the pelvic floor relaxes downward. As we exhale, the muscles of the pelvic floor draw gently in and up. One way to think about this action is to picture the center of your pelvic floor (that point midway between your genitals and anus) gently drawing in and up as you exhale. As you inhale, let this same point relax gently downward. Similarly to the belly, it is just as important to be able to let the pelvic floor relax as it is to be able to have it contract. In the following photos, my hands are placed about where the pelvic floor is located to show the subtle movement that occurs with the breath.

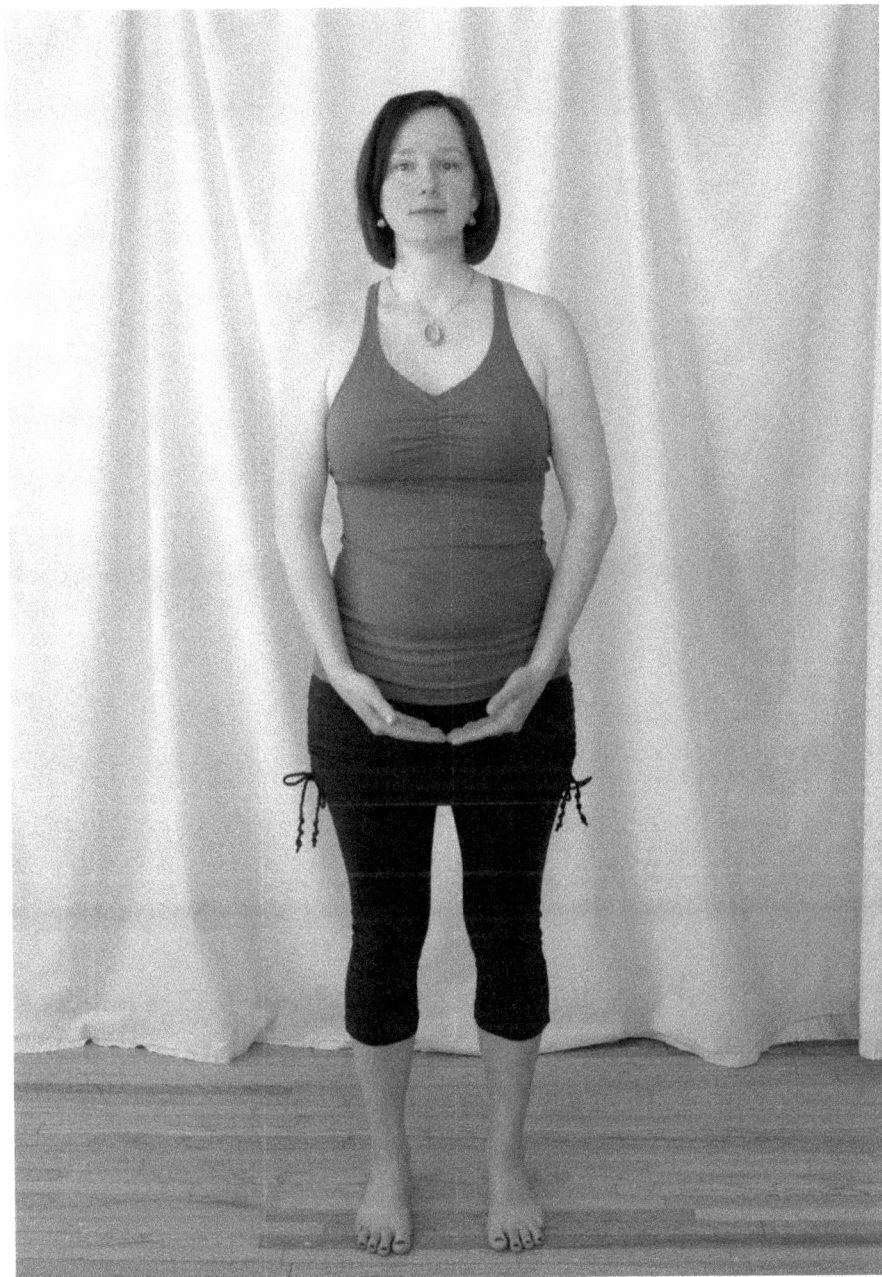

INHALE

Inhale - the breath flows all the way down into the
pelvic bowl and the pelvic floor relaxes downward.

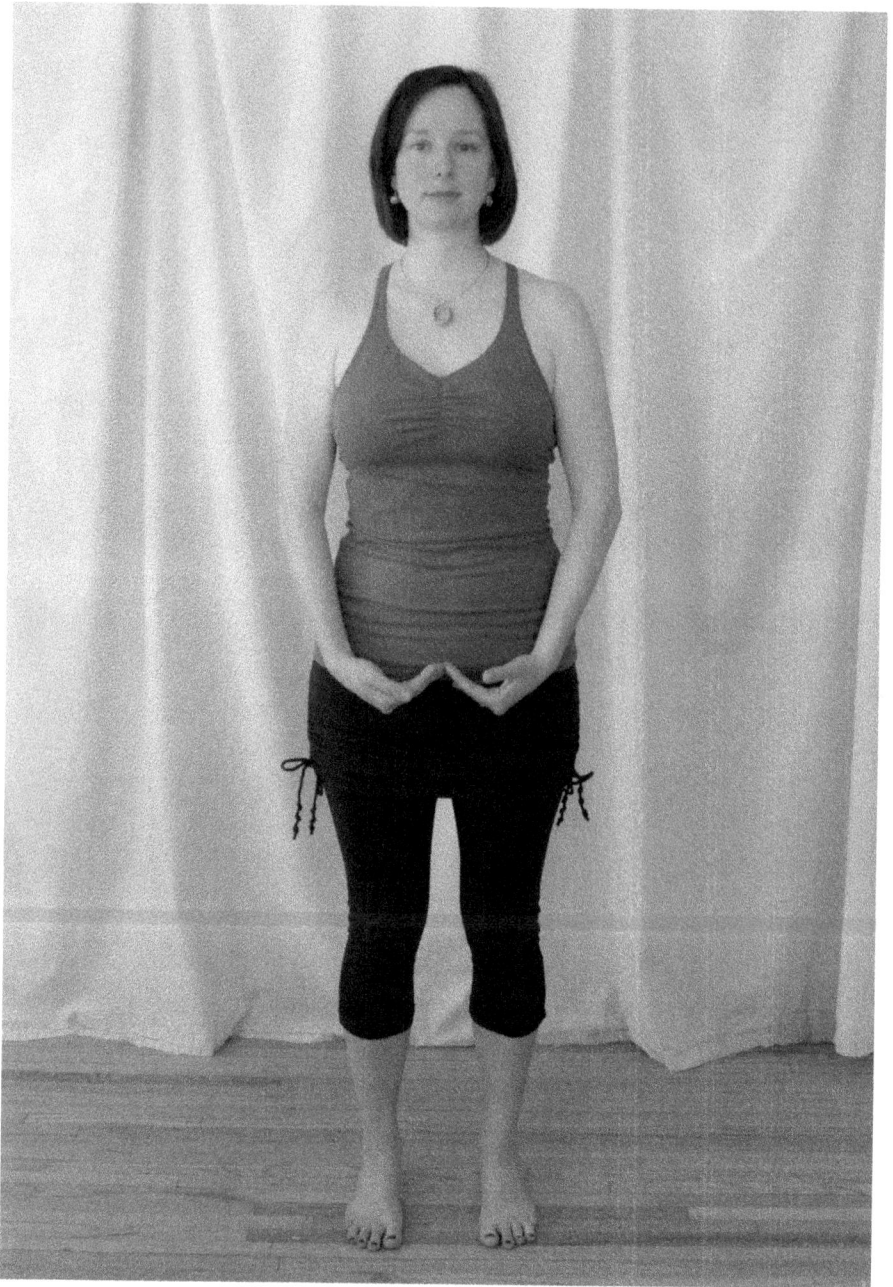

EXHALE

Exhale - the breath flows back up and out of the body and the pelvic floor rises upward. The pelvic floor is a soft sheet of overlapping muscles, so there is no pointy bit like there is with my fingers in this photo.

Let's give this awareness of the pelvic floor a try while we breathe now.

Reconnect with your tall posture as you ground down through your base and lengthen upward through the spine and crown of your head. Allow your focus to be on your breath and the subtle action of your pelvic floor. As you inhale, allow your pelvic floor to softly relax downward. As you exhale, feel your pelvic floor gently drawing in and up.

Lets take five more breaths just like that, focusing on the subtle movement of your pelvic floor.

The deep abdominal muscles and the pelvic floor muscles are considered "co-contractors" because they work best when they work together to help stabilize your spine and facilitate full breathing. Let's explore integrating the motions at the pelvic floor and the belly. With each inhale, draw your breath in and down so that it feels like your breath is flowing all the way down into the base of your pelvic bowl. As your belly gently expands outward, your pelvic floor expands downward. As you breathe out, gently draw your pelvic floor in and up, and draw your belly in and up as you exhale softly and completely.

As you inhale, allow yourself to feel a sense of expansion and spaciousness at your pelvic floor and in your belly. As you exhale, feel a sense of energetic lift from the pelvic floor, upward through your body. Feel the exhale travel upward just in front of your spine, up toward the crown of your head. Take five more breaths like that now. You may close your eyes and focus on your breath and sensations if that is helpful to you. When you feel ready, allow yourself to gently blink your eyes open.

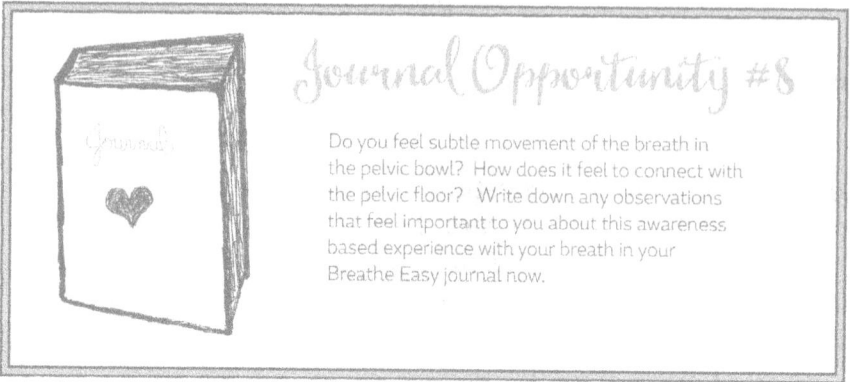

Do you feel subtle movement of the breath in the pelvic bowl? How does it feel to connect with the pelvic floor? Write down any observations that feel important to you about this awareness based experience with your breath in your Breathe Easy journal now.

If you are still having difficulty feeling the movement at the pelvic floor, don't worry. The more you tune in to the sensations of your pelvic floor and practice noticing what is happening in this area of your body, the easier this motion will become to feel. All it takes to reconnect with forgotten areas of the body is time, practice and patience. Be gentle and practice patience and kindness with yourself as you re-establish this connection.

Chapter Eight

The Intimate Relationship Between Posture and Breath

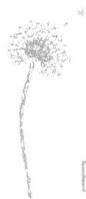

Now let's explore the intimate relationship between posture and breath. You have probably noticed that at the beginning of all of the awareness exercises we start by getting into a tall posture. Tall posture not only helps us to look younger and more attractive, but allows us to breathe more fully, too!

Let's compare how it feels to take a few deep breaths in two different postures. Use caution when moving into this first position. Let yourself slouch down, sticking your hips and head forward, allowing your chest to sink and your shoulders to slump. While you are slouched down like this, let yourself take several breaths as deeply as you are able. Notice where you feel the breath moving in your body. Does it feel like your diaphragm can move with ease? Tune in to the rate and depth of your breath. Allow yourself to take one more breath in this position.

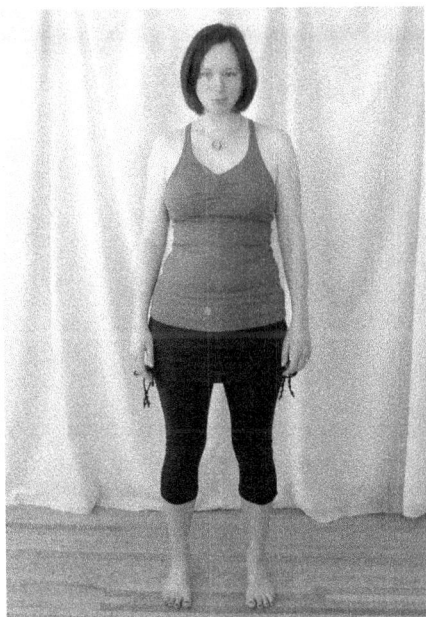

As you can see, slouchy posture makes me feel sad.

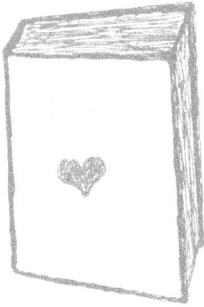

Journal Opportunity

Notice where you feel the breath moving in your body. Does it feel like your diaphragm can move with ease? Do you feel like you can breathe fully in this position? Write down any observations that feel important to you about this awareness based experience with your breath in your Breathe Easy journal now.

Notice where you feel the breath moving in your body. Does it feel like your diaphragm can move with ease? Do you feel like you can breathe fully in this position? Write down any observations that feel important to you about this awareness based experience with your breath in your Breathe Easy journal now.

Slowly and gradually begin moving back toward your tall position. Draw yourself up in a long vertical line, with your pelvis, ribcage and head all aligned, one above the other. Place one of your hands on top of your head and feel the gentle weight of your hand resting there. Allow your body to lengthen upward into the touch of your hand as the crown of your head rises upward toward the sky.

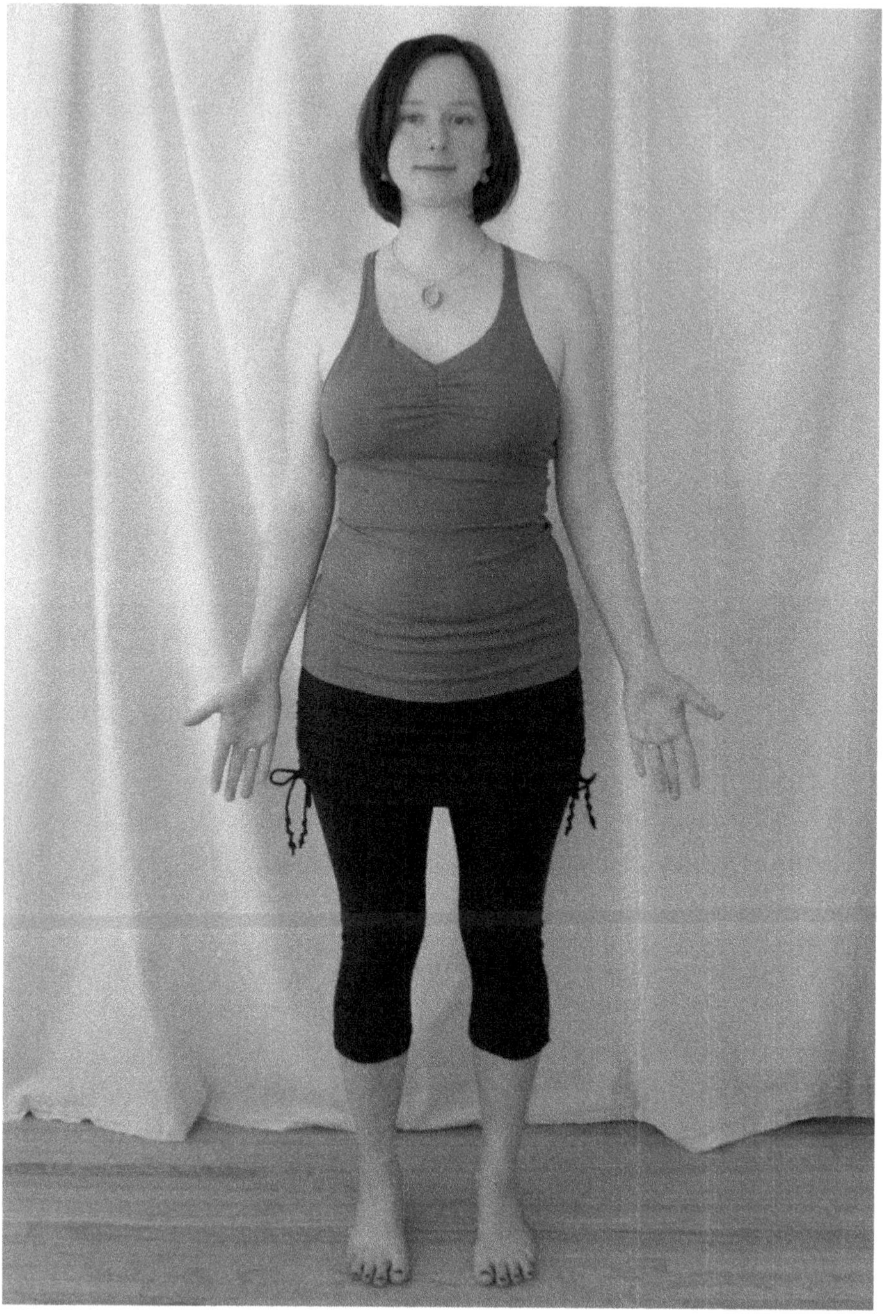

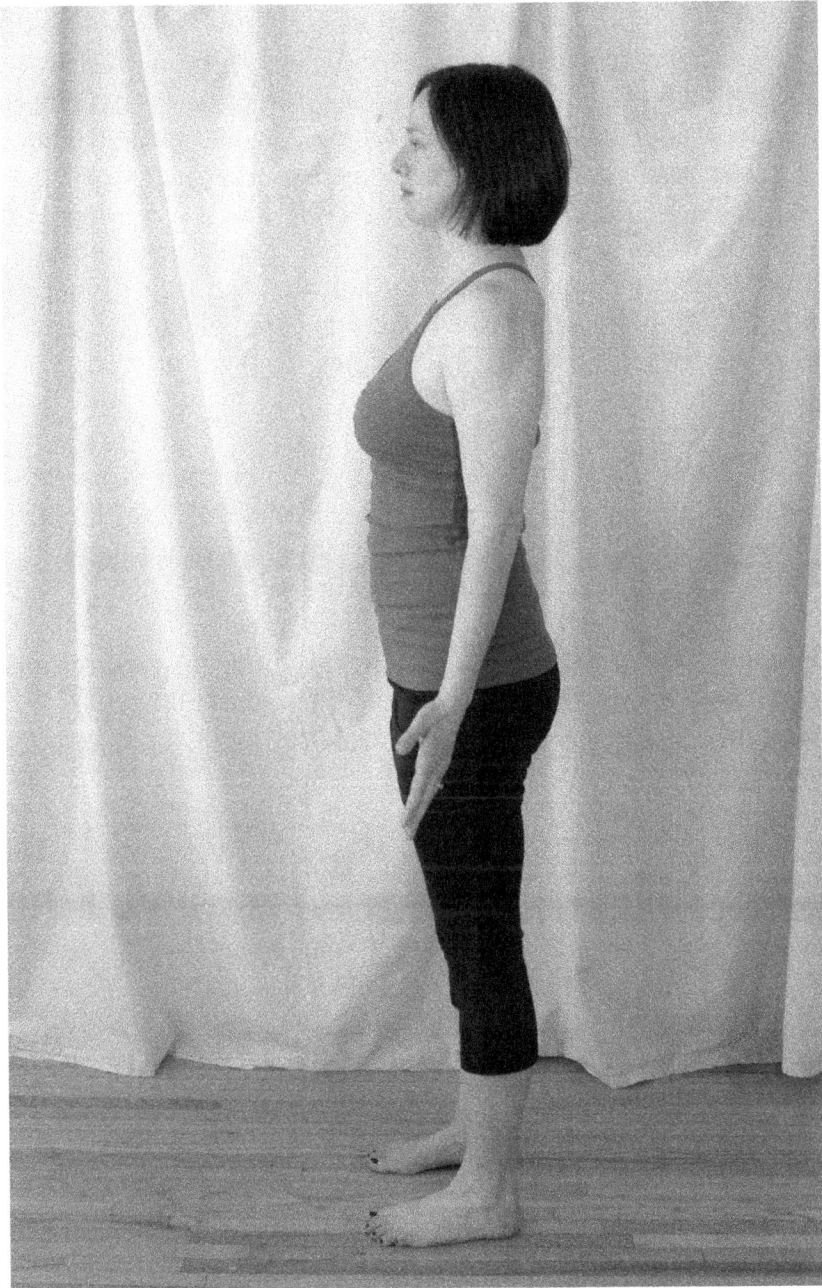

Ahhhh! That feels better! You may be able to see that I am still working toward moving my hips further backward and releasing my ribs downward. There is always something to keep you entertained in the postural/alignment world.

It is a radical choice, to actively resist against the compressive force of gravity. As gravity presses downward, we assertively rise up to meet that challenge, every day. You can allow your hand to relax down at your side now if you haven't already.

Another way to cue ourselves to maintain (or return to) upright posture is to think about raising the sternum (or breastbone) upward about half an inch to lift and open your chest, letting your collar bones stretch out long to the sides. At the same time, your back remains broad and open.

This small and subtle movement is a true act of bravery, as we resist the tendency to close off our chests and protect our hearts. By opening our chest and sharing our vulnerability with the world, we become open-hearted warriors.

The focus is on a sense of lifting and lengthening upward rather than sticking the chest out in front of you, so don't let your low ribs on the front of your body flare forward.

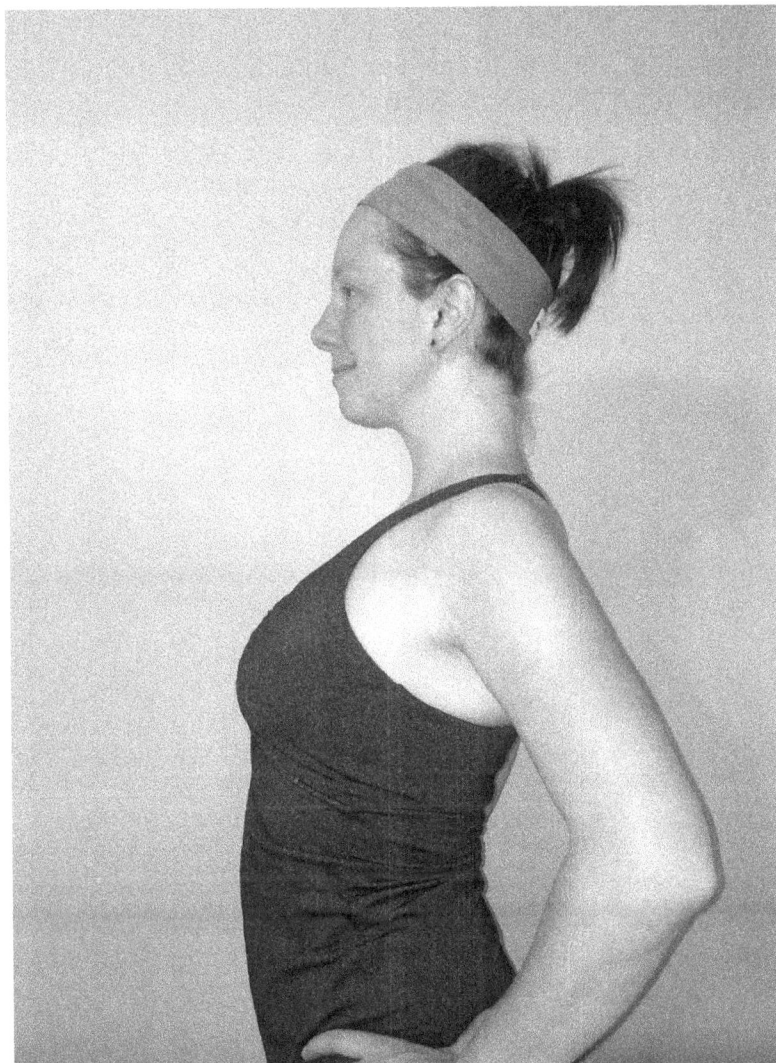

No thank you, rib flare! We often stand like this with our chest thrust forward when we are trying to stand up with "good posture". Notice the "pinch point" at the back of the body where the shirt is gathered. That is the thoraco-lumbar junction – or the point where the mid-back meets the lower back. When we flare the ribs forward we put stress at this section of our spine (that may cause pain and dysfunction at this transitional area) and change the relationship between the diaphragm and the pelvic floor in a way that interferes with their happy relationship.

Think about the low ribs in the front snuggling slightly downward and backward to prevent rib flare.

That's better! I could stand to release my front low ribs down even further than what's shown in the photo. Oh well. We are all beautiful works in progress, right?

Now, with this taller, more open posture, let yourself take several full breaths. Notice where you feel the breath moving in your body. Become aware of the rate, depth and quality of your breath. Notice which type of posture makes it easier to breathe more fully. Allow yourself to maintain this tall posture as long as you are able.

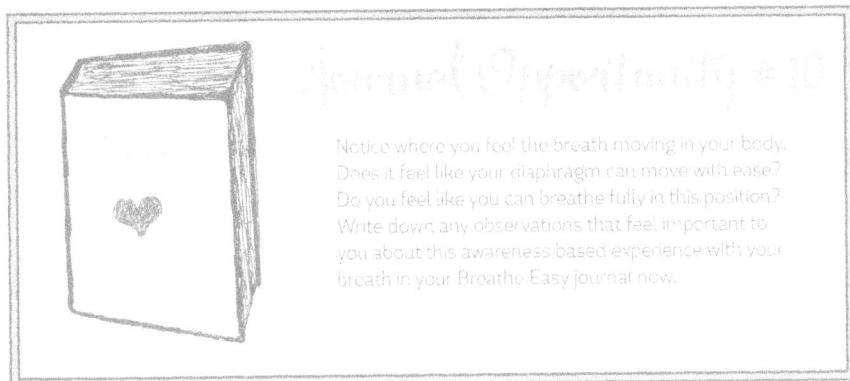

Notice where you feel the breath moving in your body. Does it feel like your diaphragm can move with ease? Do you feel like you can breathe fully in this position? Write down any observations that feel important to you about this awareness based experience with your breath in your Breathe Easy journal now.

Do not be discouraged if it feels challenging to keep a tall posture. Posture, like breath, is an awareness-based practice. When you notice that you are slouching or feeling compressed, gently remind yourself to lengthen upward and open your chest.

If you are too tired to lengthen, it could be a sign that it may be a good time to lie down on your back with something under your knees or with your legs up, to rest for a while. This gives your postural muscles a break from working against gravity in that same old way. This is a good place to mention that your breath practice can also be done quite comfortably and successfully in a number of positions. Some examples are shown below.*

Lie on back with bolster or pillow under knees

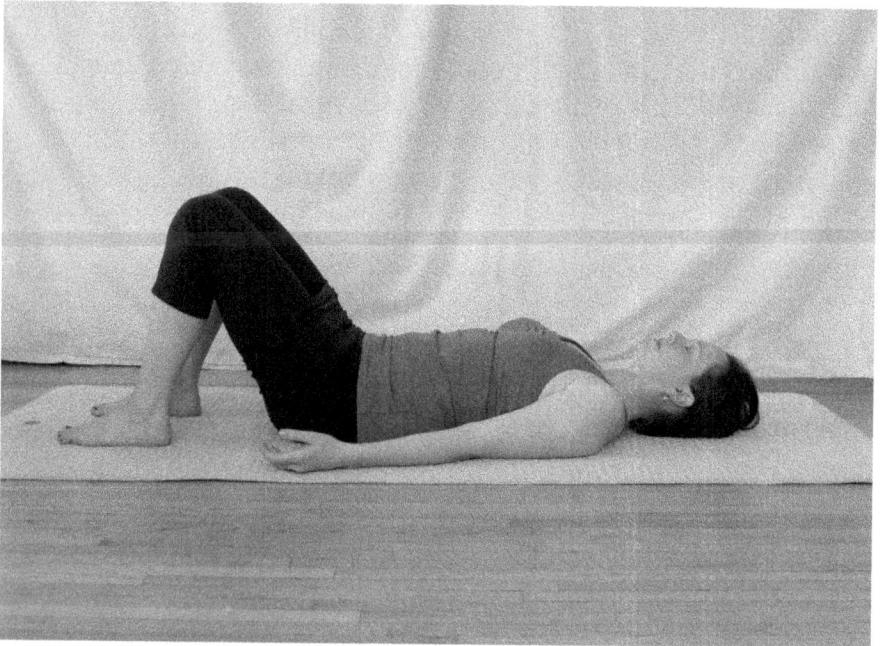

Lie on back with knees bent and feet on the floor

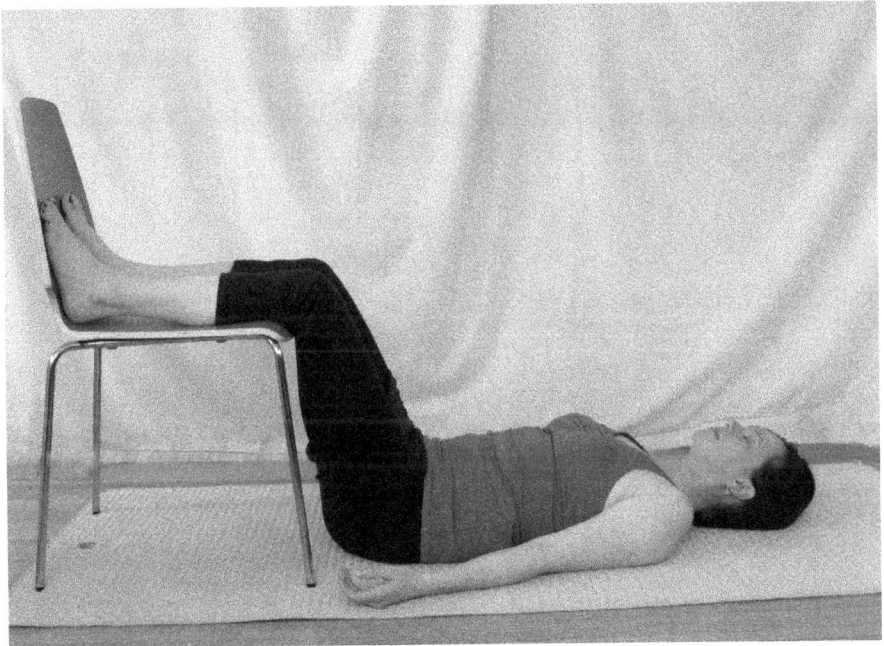

Lie on back with legs on seat of chair

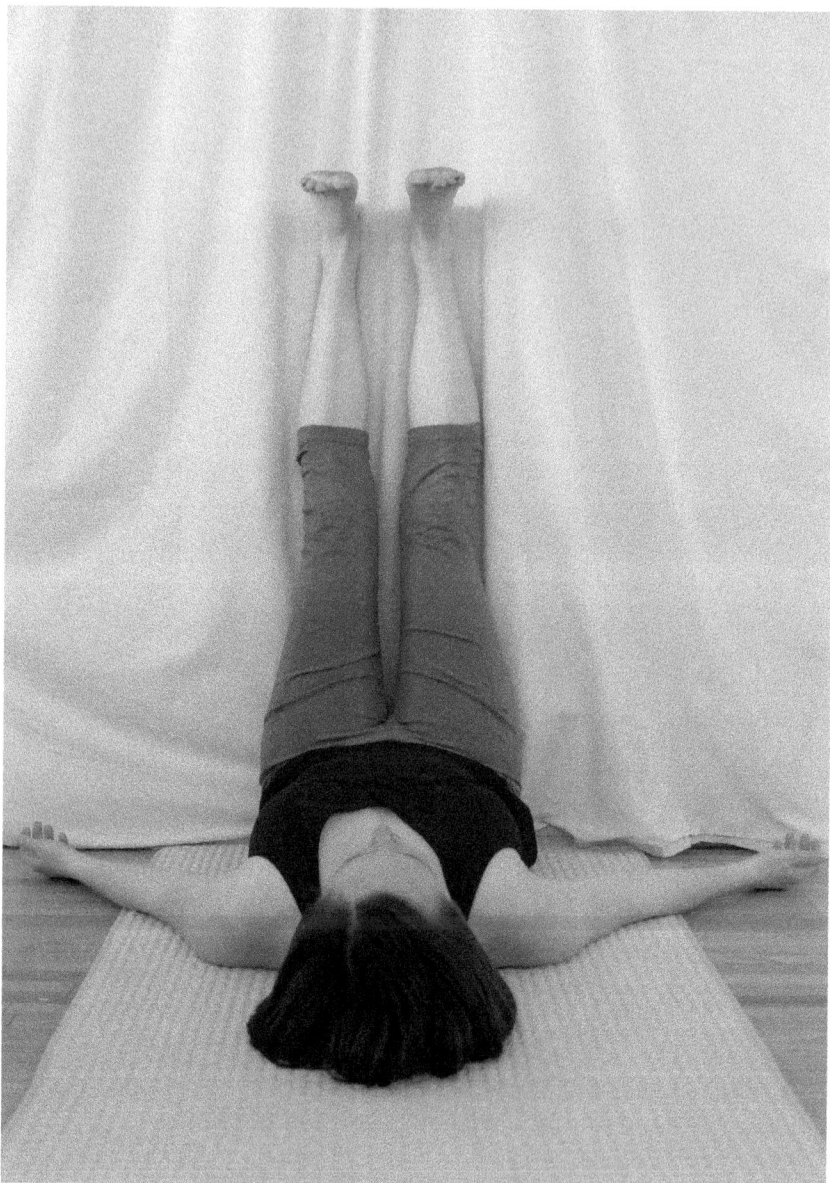

Lie on back with legs up wall

*You could also place a pillow beneath your head if that helps you to feel relaxed and comfortable or use a bolster or pillow under your head and shoulders to help your ribs release downward. Please explore any options that facilitate your comfort and allow you to deeply relax during your breathing practice.

When you notice that you are slouching or feeling compressed, it could also be a good reminder to change your position entirely. Maybe it's time to get up and move. Dance, take a walk or enjoy any other fun and novel movements that inspire you and pique your interest. We aren't intended to hold a static position for a long time, even an excellent upright one. If you are in any position for too long, eventually it can start feeling rigid and held. Just like we talked about with the abdominal wall, we don't want to be in a rigid holding pattern. We want to develop and maintain fluidity in our body and our breath.

Congratulate yourself when you begin to notice things like your posture and your breath. Once you begin to notice your posture and breath you have already won. You can only begin to change habits once you are aware of them.

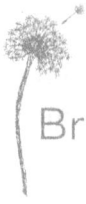

Chapter Nine

Breathing Into the Back of the Body

Another dramatic change that we can begin to make right now, is to begin breathing in all three dimensions. We can begin using the lung space on the sides and back of the body in addition to what we have already explored on the front. As we briefly touched on before, there is lung space on all sides of your body. We typically don't think about breathing into our sides and back, unless we are taught that this type of breath is even a possibility and are then shown how.

Let's begin with feeling the breath on the back of the body. Begin to focus your attention on feeling the breath as it travels in and down along the back of your body.

With each inhale, feel the breath moving in and down along the channel just forward of your spine all the way until it reaches the tip of your tailbone. As you exhale, feel the breath trace that same path back up and out of the body as it leaves through the nostrils.

With each inhale, feel a sense of expansion between your shoulder blades and a general broadening across the whole back body. With each exhale, feel a gentle sense of lift from your hip bones, upward through your waist along the spine. Inhale and feel the space at the base of the ribcage on the back of your body broadening and expanding. Exhale and feel this same area soften and release.

Allow your eyes to close if this helps you tune in to your breath. Take five more breaths focusing on the sensation of the breath in the back body. When you feel ready, gently open your eyes.

It can be challenging at first to feel the breath as it moves through the sides and back of the body. Many people find it helpful to have some sort of hands-on or tactile feedback when first attempting to feel the breath in these areas. This feedback can be achieved independently, or by working with a partner.

If you are working independently, take a moment to find some clear wall space to lean against. Come to a tall standing position with your back against the wall and your knees bent slightly.

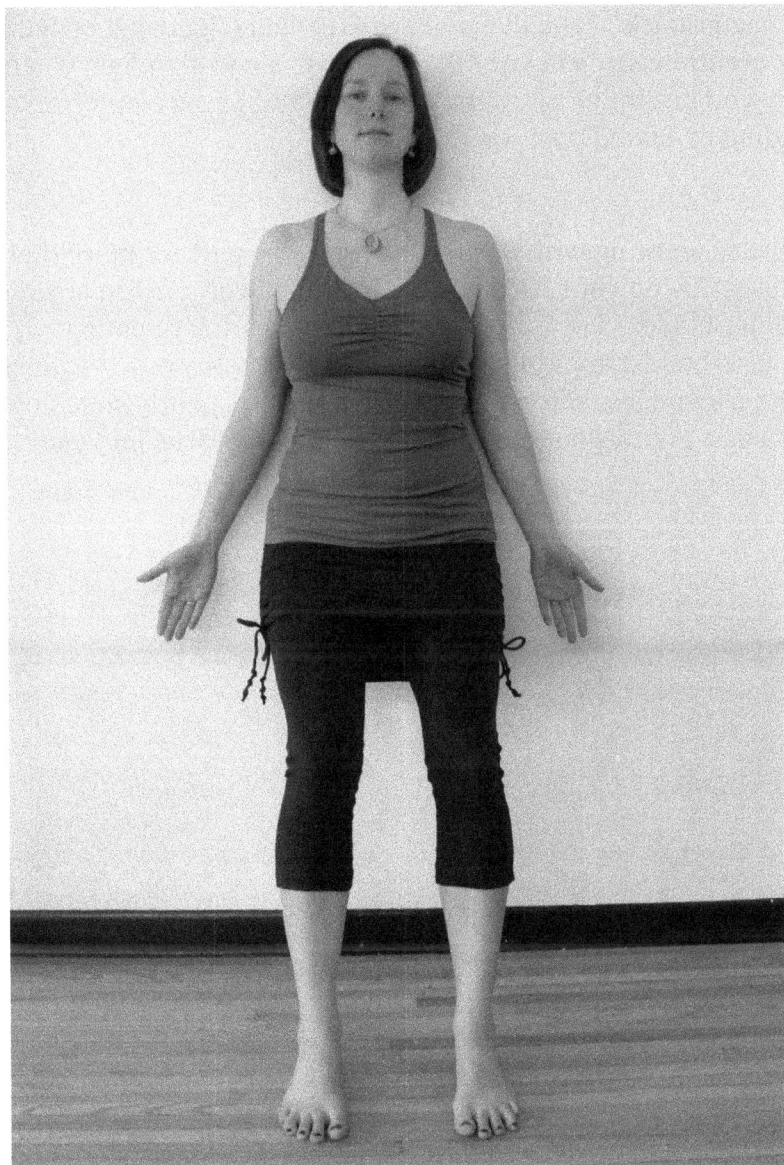

Throughout this process, allow yourself to breathe in and out at your own pace. When you feel ready, begin to take some full breaths into the back of your body. Feel the area where your back touches the wall expanding and filling with your breath. On your inhale, gently feel the breath fill your back so that it broadens and presses against the wall. On your exhale, feel your back soften. Let your neck and jaw soften. Feel your shoulders gently slide down your back. Take five more breaths here, focusing on feeling your breath moving in your back, against the wall. When you feel ready you can move away from the wall and find a comfortable standing or seated position.

If you are working with a partner, have your partner place their hands gently on your back, just inside the lower portion of your shoulder blades. Focus on sending your breath into your partner's hands, thinking about filling them with your breath. Let your neck and jaw soften. Feel your shoulders gently slide down your back. Allow yourself to take two more breaths into your back body.

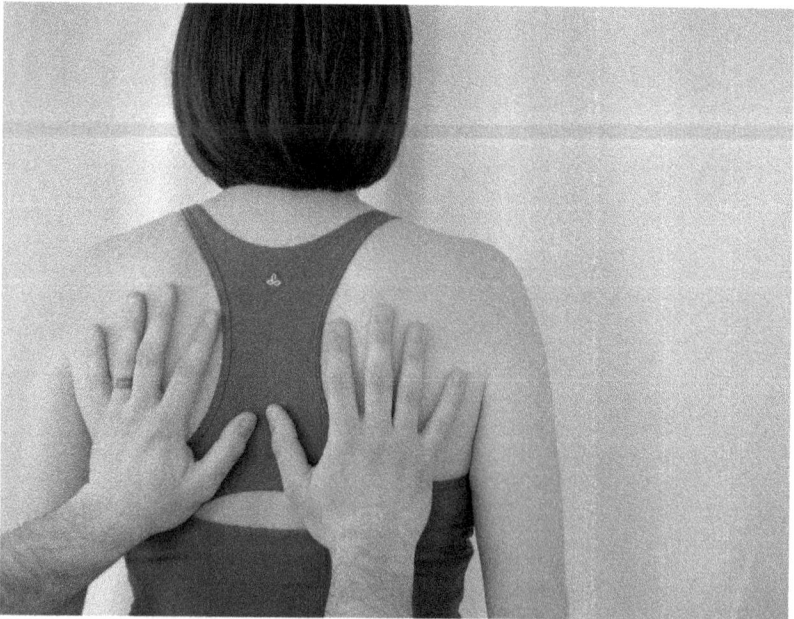

INHALE; the back gently broadens and your partner's hands spread slightly apart

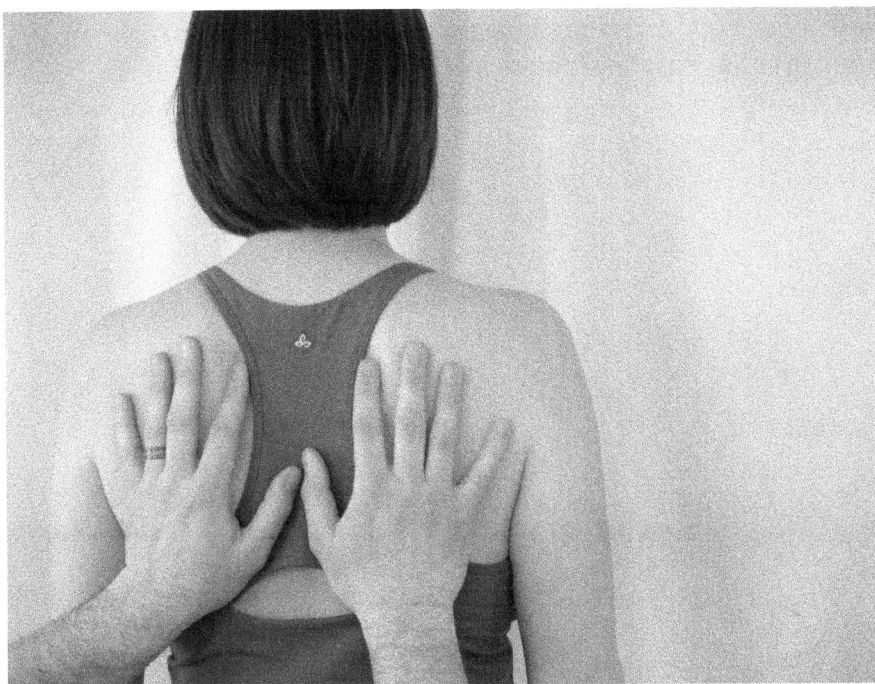

EXHALE; the back gently releases and your partner's hands draw closer together

If you have chosen to work with a partner today, you can reverse roles and then talk with each other about your experience.

Journal Opportunity #11

Do you feel your breath moving on the back side of your body? Did it help you to use feedback from the wall or from the hands of a partner? Write down any observations that feel important to you about this awareness based experience with your breath in your Breathe Easy journal now.

Do you feel your breath moving on the back side of your body? Did it help you to use feedback from the wall or from the hands of a partner? Write down any observations that feel important to you about your awareness based experience with your breath in your Breathe Easy journal now.

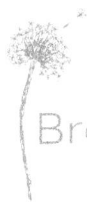

Chapter Ten

Breathing Into the Sides of the Body

Now let's take our awareness to the sides of the body. Noticing the movement of the breath along the sides of the body can feel daunting at first because the movement is so subtle. Using feedback from your own hands or the hands of a partner can help you to feel your breath, especially when you are first starting out.

If you are working independently, place your hands so that they wrap around the sides of your ribcage with your thumb pointing backward. Try to place your hands up as high as you comfortably can on your ribs.

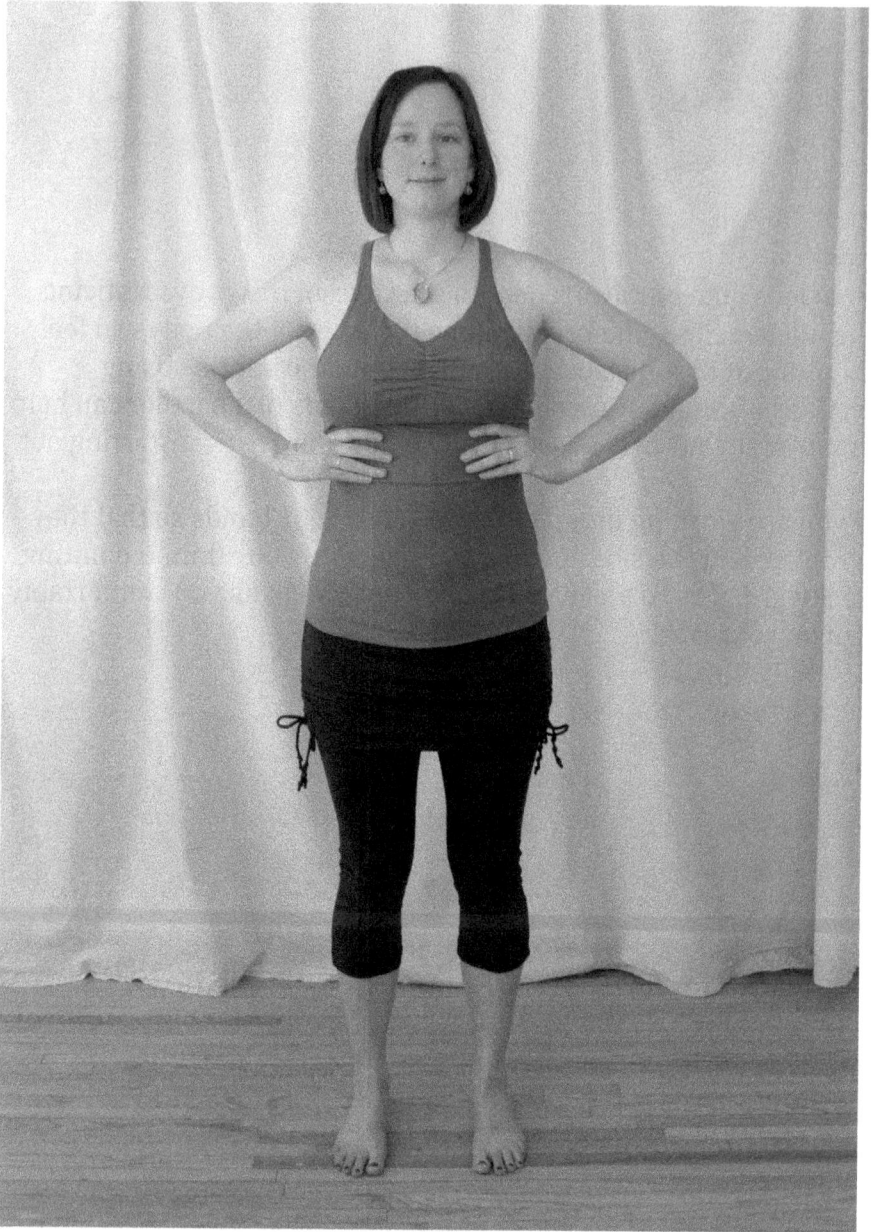

INHALE; feel the ribs expand out toward the sides,
moving into the hands

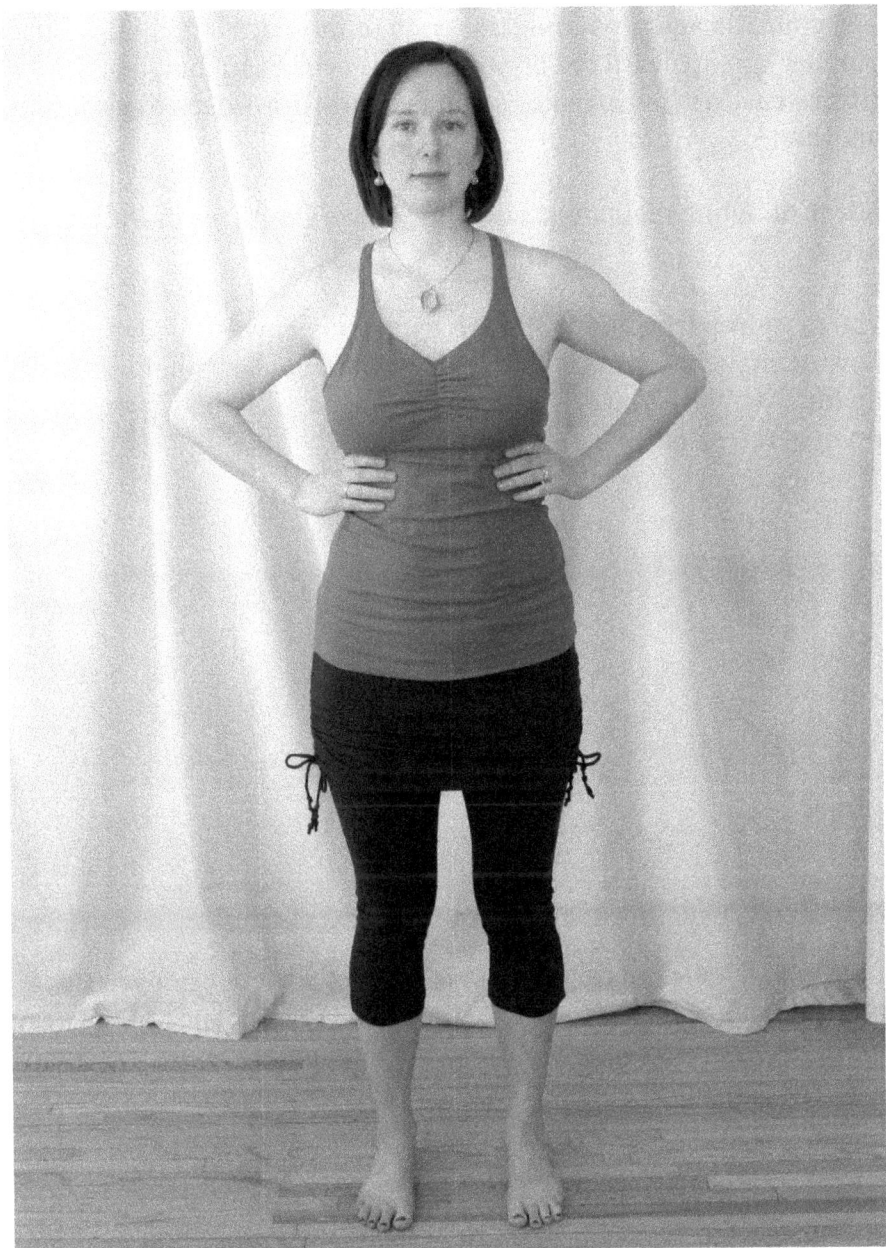

EXHALE; feel the ribs, and the hands, gently moving back toward the midline

If you are working with a partner, have your partner place their hands in that same space under your arms. With each breath in, feel your ribcage expanding out wide to the sides and filling your partner's hands with the breath. With each breath out, feel the ribs release as your partner's hands gently draw back toward one another.

Focus on filling the hands with your breath for three more breaths.

You or your partner can let your arms relax down at your sides now or shake them out if that feels good to you after holding them up for a while. If you are working with a partner today, you can reverse roles and share your experience.

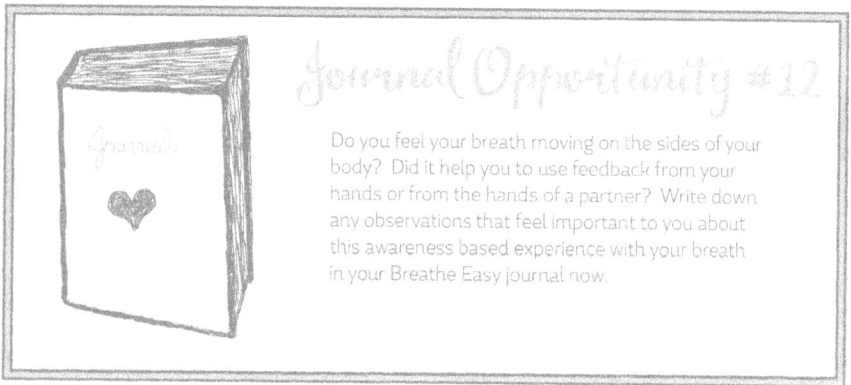

Journal Opportunity #12

Do you feel your breath moving on the sides of your body? Did it help you to use feedback from your hands or from the hands of a partner? Write down any observations that feel important to you about this awareness based experience with your breath in your Breathe Easy journal now.

Do you feel your breath moving on the sides of your body? Did it help you to use feedback from your hands or the hands of a partner? Write down any observations that feel important to you about this awareness based experience with your breath in your Breathe Easy journal now.

It may be difficult to feel the breath moving in the sides because the ribcage has become stiff from lack of movement. Most humans don't move the ribcage in a way that encourages it to keep any sort of flexibility. If you are feeling like your whole ribcage is stiff and it is challenging to breathe into the full space of the lungs on all sides of the body, I invite you to try the stretches shown below. After resting and breathing in these positions, try the back and side body focused breathing exercises again and notice if it feels like you can access those areas with greater ease. As always, if these stretches don't feel good in your body, please stop doing them until you can get more clarification about how to modify them so that they are safe for you and do feel good in your body.

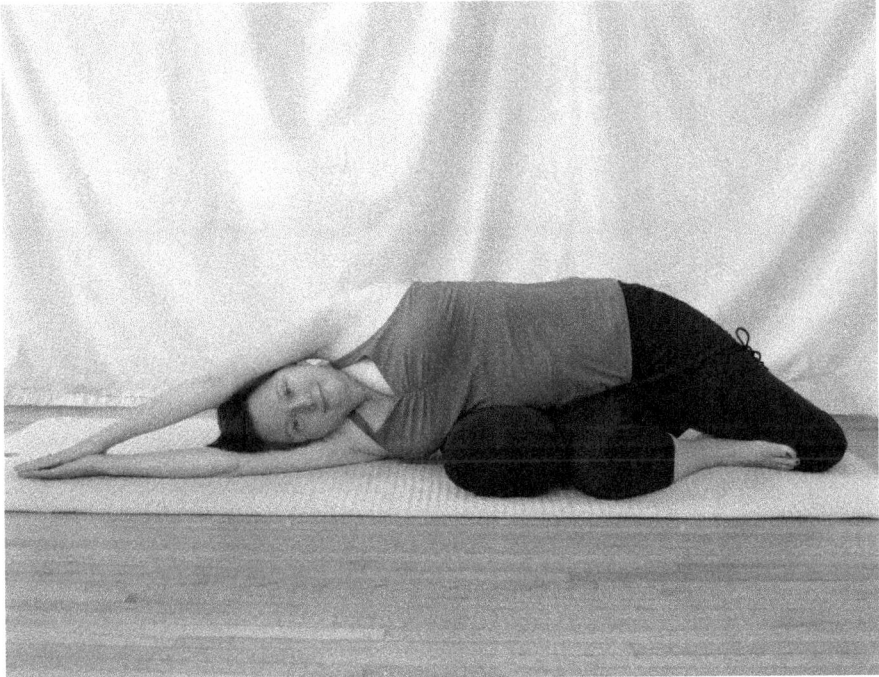

Side bend over a bolster or stacked pillows. Focus your breathing into the top side of the ribcage as it expands in this position.

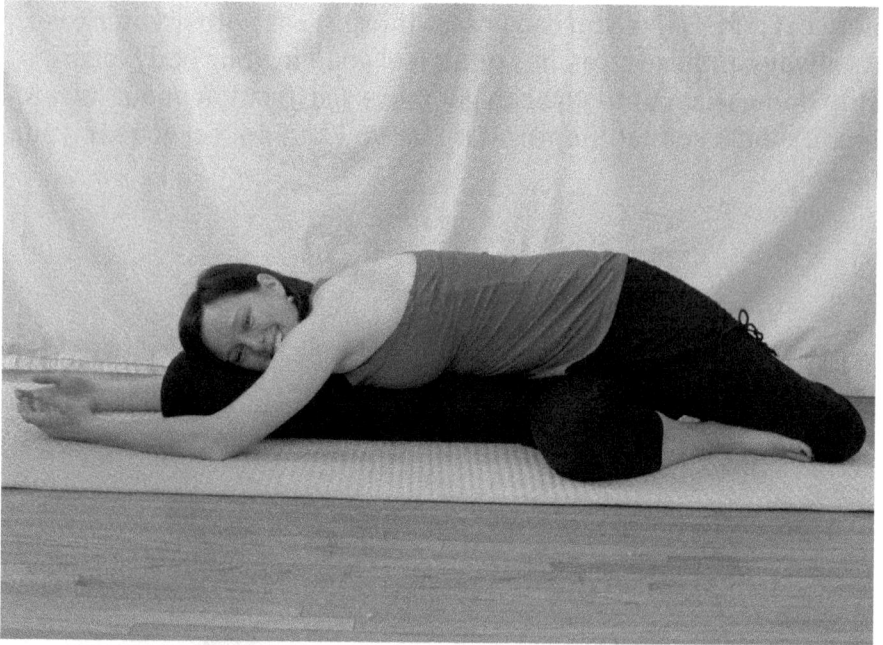

Rotation over a bolster or stacked pillows. Focus your breathing into the top side of the ribcage as it expands in this position.

If you would like a bit more instruction about how to get into these positions and where to focus your breathing while you are practicing them, please check out the video tutorials on working with a bolster in a side bend and rotation at backinbody.com under the video tutorials menu tab.

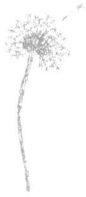

Chapter Eleven

3D Breath – Breathing In All Directions

Now that you have connected with the breath on the sides and back of your body, let's incorporate several of the elements we played with earlier.

This is where things can feel like a lot to integrate when you're first getting started. I encourage you to use tender loving patience and give yourself permission to integrate these components at your own pace. It will all come together with regular practice and time.

Allow yourself to find your tall posture, lengthening and lifting upward.

Let your awareness be drawn to your breath. Feel the breath as it moves in and out through your nostrils. Allow yourself to observe your breath as it is right now without changing anything.

Become aware of the rate of your breath, whether it feels fast or slow.

Notice the depth of your breath, whether it feels shallow or deep.

Check in with the quality of your breath, noticing whether it is flowing smoothly or has rough edges.

Notice if there is any sound associated with your breath.

Are there are any emotions or feelings associated with this experience of your breath? Let yourself feel what is there without the need to get into any story around it.

Allow yourself to suspend any judgment about whether the way you are breathing is "good" or "bad" and let your self be fully present with what is. Notice where you feel your breath moving in your body. Gradually invite your breath to become more full and deep.

As you breathe in, allow your belly to gently soften and expand outward and downward. As you breathe out, gently draw your belly inward and upward to press out any stale air that may be lingering in the lower parts of your lungs. Allow the breath to begin to flow more deeply. With each inhale, draw your breath in and down so that it feels like your breath is flowing all the way down into the base of your pelvic bowl. As your belly gently expands outward, your pelvic floor expands downward. As you breathe out, gently draw your pelvic floor in and up, and draw your belly in and up as you exhale softly and completely.

As you take a breath in, visualize your breath traveling in and down through your nostrils, chest and abdomen, until it fills your pelvic bowl. As you breathe out, visualize the breath traveling up and out through your abdomen and chest, then exiting through your nostrils, as you feel a sense of energetic lift from the pelvic floor, upward through your body - traveling along the channel just forward of your spine. With each inhale, feel the breath flowing in and down - filling the body from the pelvic bowl, up though the abdomen, ribcage and chest. With each exhale, feel the softening - letting go of what you no longer need. Continue breathing in this slow smooth fashion.

Draw your awareness around to the sensations at the back of your body. With each inhale, feel the breath moving in and down along the channel just forward of your spine all the way until it reaches the tip of your tailbone. As you exhale, feel the breath trace that same path back up and out of the body as it leaves through the nostrils. With each inhale, feel a sense of expansion between your shoulder blades and a general broadening across the whole back body. With each exhale, feel a gentle sense of lift from your hip bones, upward through your waist along the spine.

72

Allow yourself to draw your awareness around to the sides of your body. With each breath in, notice a sense of expansion under your arms. With each breath out, feel the ribcage gently releasing. Inhale, feel your ribcage expanding out wide to the sides. Exhale, feel your ribcage soften.

Draw your awareness now to the breath as it flows freely on all sides of the body. With each inhale, feel the breath flowing in and down - filling the body from the pelvic bowl, up though the abdomen, ribcage and chest on all sides of the body. With each exhale, feel the breath traveling up and out, as your pelvic floor, belly, sides and back gently draw inward and upward.

With each inhale, draw the breath in and down all the way to the base of your pelvic bowl, feeling your pelvic floor soften, your belly, sides and back of your body expanding in all directions With each exhale, softening - letting go of what you no longer need. As you continue breathing in this slow smooth fashion, your body and mind become more and more deeply relaxed.

Allow yourself to take five more breaths this way at your own pace, feeling a sense of expansion and spaciousness as you inhale... and a sense of release as you exhale. With each breath in, feel yourself filling the container of your body with fresh air. With each breath out, feel the softening of your shoulders, neck and jaw. Feel free to close your eyes and focus on your breath and sensations if that is helpful to you. When you feel ready, allow your eyes to gently open.

Journal Opportunity #13

How does it feel to breathe into the fullness of the container of your body? What thoughts or feelings do you have at this point? Write down any observations that feel important to you about this awareness based experience with your breath in your Breathe Easy journal now.

How does it feel to breathe into the fullness of the container of your body? What thoughts or feelings do you have at this point? Write down any observations that feel important to you about this awareness based experience with your breath in your Breathe Easy journal now.

Chapter Twelve

Rib Movement, Bucket Handles and Calipers...Oh My!

Of course, things aren't complex enough yet, right? The human body and its functions are definitely gloriously complex. In the spirit of beautiful complexity, we're going to add another layer to our concept of ribcage movement. The ribs go through some very subtle motions with each breath in and out. We will explore these movements using our arms as a visual guide of how one pair of our ribs will move as we breathe.

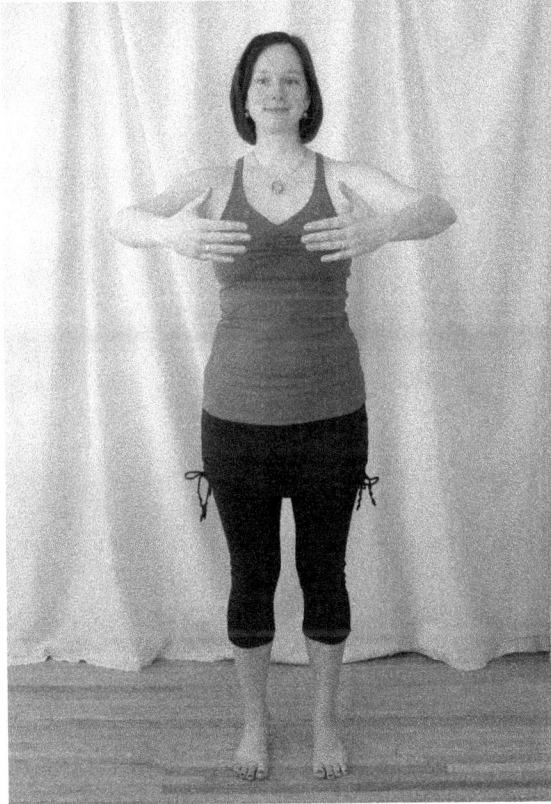

Raise your arms out in front of you, making them into a circle shape with some slight space between your hands. Picture your body representing your spine, and each arm as a rib on either side of your ribcage. Your sternum, or breastbone would be in the open space between your hands.

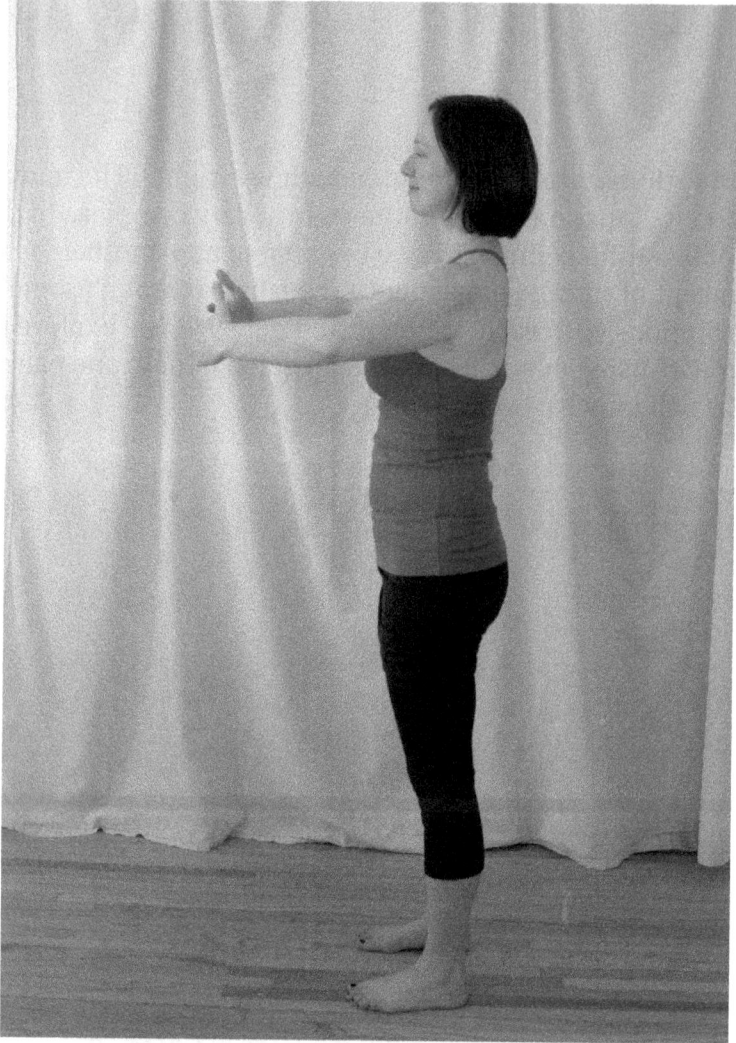

When you breathe, your ribs go through two different types of motions at the same time - caliper motion and bucket handle motion. Lets take a look at caliper motion first.

When observing caliper motion, you notice that as you take a breath in, your chest expands front to back and side to side. When you breathe out, your chest gently contracts and draws back as your breath leaves the lungs. As you inhale, allow your hands to move forward slightly further away from your chest. As you exhale, allow your hands to move back toward their starting position. Take 3 breaths at your own pace, moving the arms in this fashion and tuning in to the movement at your ribcage. You can let your arms relax at your sides when you are done playing with this movement.

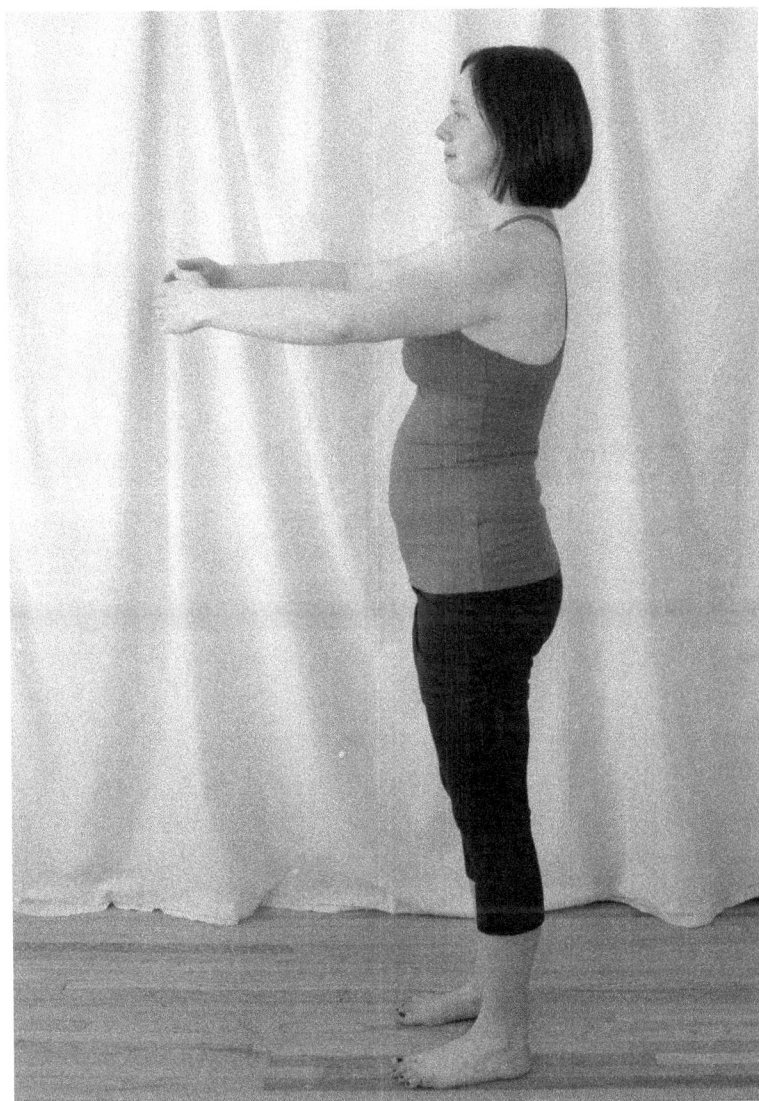

INHALE

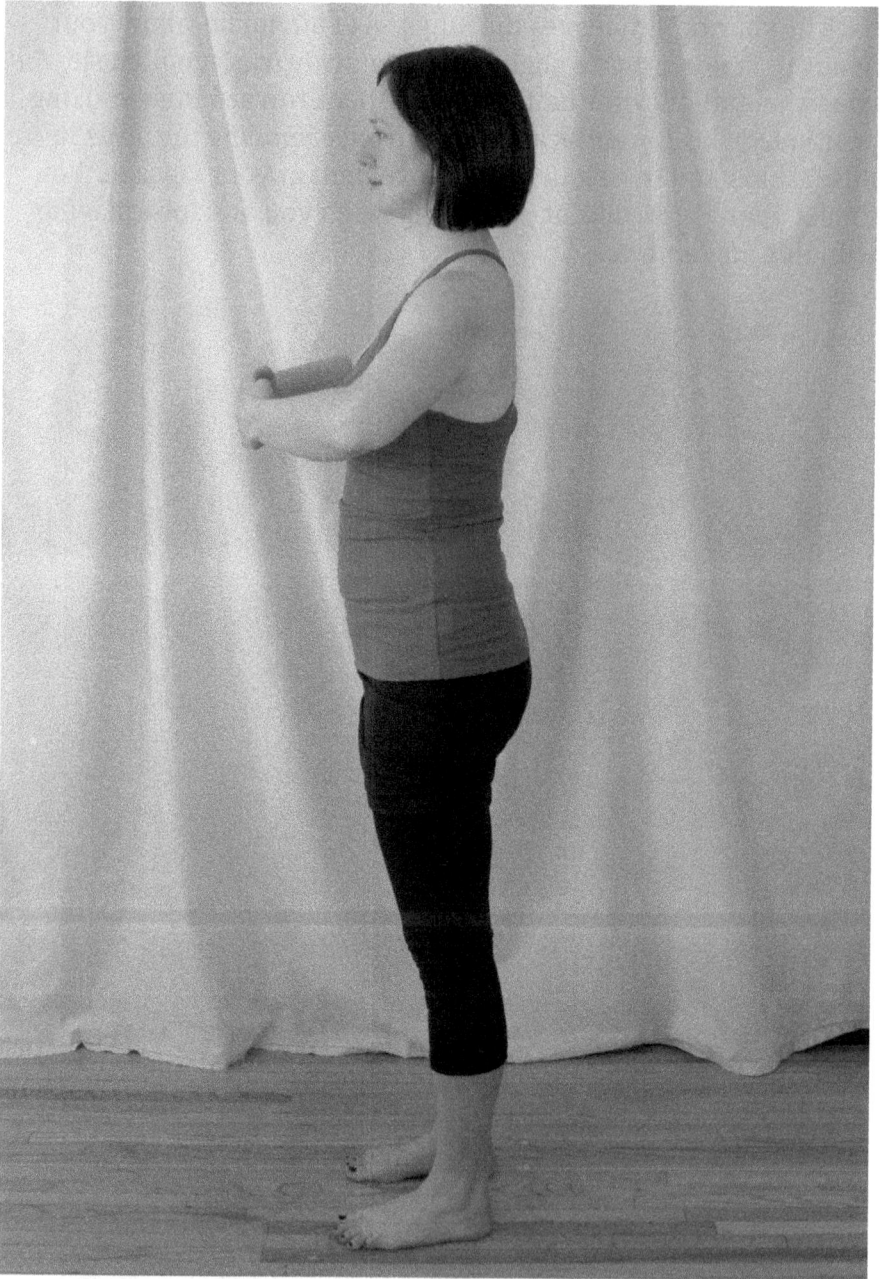

EXHALE

Now lets explore bucket handle movement. When we inhale, our ribs flare slightly upward in a motion similar to raising our elbows while keeping the hands about where they are. When we exhale, our ribs draw gently back downward, as if our elbows were to gently lower back to their starting position.

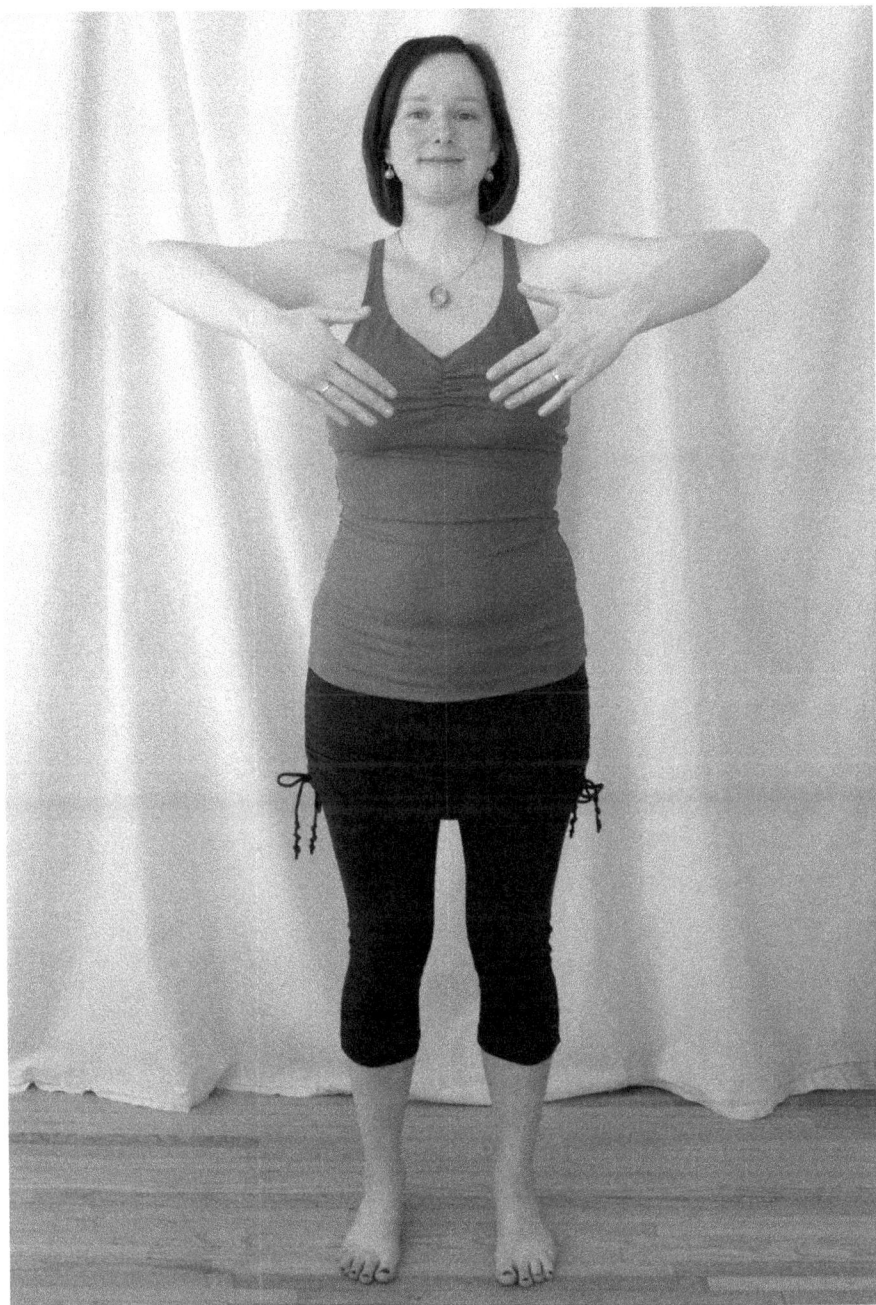

INHALE

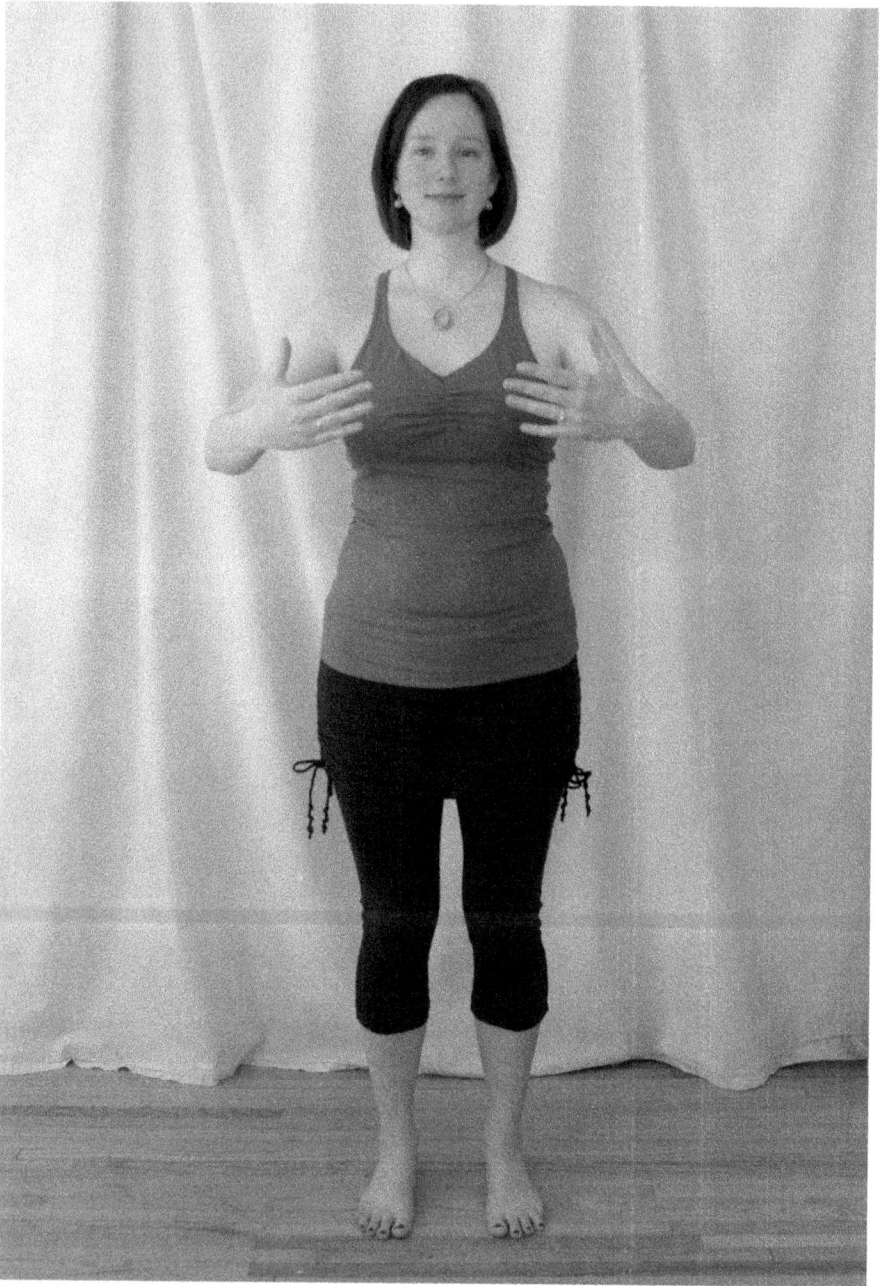

EXHALE

Allow yourself to take three full breaths at your own pace while you move your arms in this bucket handle motion and tune in to this movement at your ribcage. When you are done exploring this motion, let your arms relax at your sides.

Sometimes, an individual rib will become stuck, and won't be able to move through the full range of caliper or bucket handle motion. This would be considered a segmental restriction (affecting one specific segment) rather than a global restriction (general tightness throughout the whole ribcage) like we talked about when using the stretches over the bolster to increase ribcage mobility. It can be very helpful to visit a Doctor of Chiropractic (or another healthcare practitioner who is well trained in gentle and specific joint mobilization) to have your body checked for segmental restrictions and then adjusted to restore motion to those specific segments. Removing segmental rib and thoracic (mid back) restrictions through chiropractic adjusting can allow for more freedom of motion through the ribcage in a full deep breath pattern.

Those two motions, caliper and bucket handle motion, don't happen in isolation... they happen together at the same time. At this point, lets take three breaths combining these motions and notice the movement at your ribcage as we do so. As we inhale, the hands move forward, and the elbows flare upward. As we exhale, our hands gently move backward and our elbows lower downward. Take two more breaths like that. Let your arms relax down to the sides.

As we acknowledge the full shape of our body and expand our awareness to include all sides of our body moving fully with the breath, we begin to move our consciousness down from its common space in our heads and faces on the front side of our body. As our breath and awareness move more fully into the body, we begin to experience what it feels like to inhabit our center. The more you practice intentional breathing, the more refined your awareness of your body will become. It is fascinating to discover the messages and wisdom of the body when we become centered and still enough to listen. The breath is our vehicle to find that stillness and to begin this exploration of the body's way of knowing.

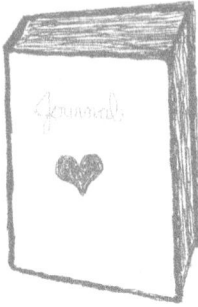

Journal Opportunity #14

Do you feel the subtle caliper motion at the ribs?
Do you feel the bucket handle motion at the ribs?
How does it feel to have your breath flowing fully
into and out of your body? Write down any
observations that feel important to you about
this awareness based experience with your breath
in your Breathe Easy journal now.

Do you feel the subtle caliper motion at the ribs? Do you feel the bucket handle motion at the ribs? How does it feel to have your breath flowing fully into and out of your body? Write down any observations that feel important to you about this awareness based experience with your breath in your Breathe Easy journal now.

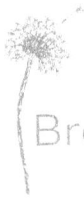

Chapter Thirteen

Breathing Into Your Head Space

Now let's take our awareness of the breath into an area that may seem like a strange place to notice movement - the space inside our heads. We have explored this theme of a sense of spaciousness and expansion on the inhale and a sense of lift, of drawing in and up on the exhale at many areas of the body. Now let's apply this same awareness to the subtle sensations within our head space. Allow your breath to gradually deepen. Begin to draw your awareness to the space between your ears and behind your eyes.

With each breath in, feel an increasing sense of spaciousness and expansion within your head space. As you exhale, allow yourself to feel a gentle sense of lift, upward through the crown of your head - as if you are a whale softly spraying water up out of your spout. Inhale, feel the space between your ears broadening and your eyes softening. Exhale, feeling the crown of the head floating lightly upward. Allow yourself to take five more breaths at your own pace, feeling this spaciousness on your inhale, and sense of release on your exhale. Feel free to close your eyes and focus on your breath and sensations if that is helpful to you. As you feel ready, allow yourself to gently blink your eyes open.

Check in with how you feel right now.

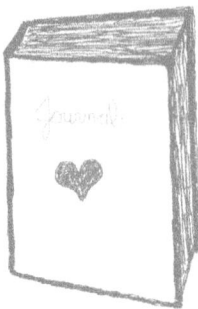

Journal Opportunity #15

How does it feel to bring your awareness into your head space? Do you feel a sense of expansion in the space between your ears and behind your eyes on your inhale? As you exhale is there anything you can feel yourself releasing? Write down any observations that feel important to you about this awareness based experience with your breath in your Breathe Easy journal now.

How does it feel to bring your awareness into your head space? Do you feel a sense of expansion in the space between your ears and behind your eyes on your inhale? As you exhale, is there anything you can feel yourself releasing? Write down any observations that feel important to you about this awareness based experience with your breath in your Breathe Easy journal now.

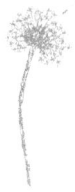

Chapter Fourteen

Why Breathing Matters –
Words and Traditions

Let's look at the breath in the context of why intentional breathing is important and what breathing more fully can do for us in our daily life. Our breath is the very first and very last thing we experience during life in our fabulous body. Those first and last breaths are loaded with drama and attention, but usually we completely forget about our breath during the majority of our life in between - unless we become sick and are having difficulty breathing.

Words and language choices can provide some rich context for the importance of the breath. The alternate words for inhale and exhale are loaded with meaning... they are INSPIRE and EXPIRE! Inspiration means being filled with the presence of Spirit! In Judeo-Christian traditions, the breath of God is what brings life to humankind. Inspiration is our breath in, or drawing in of spirit at the beginning of life and expiration is the departure of the spirit... the final exhale at the end of our lives in our physical body. In the yogic tradition the Sanskrit word prana is used to describe both the breath and the spirit, as they are fully and completely linked. Many other religious and spiritual traditions have breath and spirit intimately connected through language choices as well.

There are also many phrases used in day to day conversation that reveal some conventional wisdom about the importance of the breath. Have you ever heard someone describe a more relaxed or spacious feeling schedule as allowing for more breathing room? How about the idea that we take a deep breath to prepare for a challenge or to improve our focus? Or taking ten deep breaths to move from a reactive state when angry so we can think more clearly and calmly before taking any action? When we think about the significance of the breath, it seems compelling to begin to honor the breath as part of a life long practice.

The way our breath affects how our body works also provides many good reasons to begin breathing more fully.

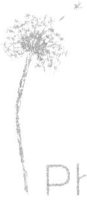

Chapter Fifteen

Why Breathing Matters –
Physiology (How the Body Works)

There is a Sanskrit proverb that states: For breath is life, and if you breathe well you will live long on earth. This link between breathing well and healthy outcomes is not just a thing of proverbs. It is well established that full intentional breathing has a very dramatic impact on how our body works!

Our breath is one of very few ways we can quickly and directly make changes to our physiology. When we breathe using a full, steady breath pattern, we are giving a break to our hard working heart and cardiovascular system. Our heart rate slows and our blood pressure lowers. Our body can focus on repair functions, like healing the wear and tear that comes along with constant use.

The alternating change in pressure between the abdomen and chest that happens when we breathe with our diaphragm creates a pumping action that helps return blood from the inferior vena cava (a large vein bringing oxygen poor blood back from the lower body) to the heart. The blood can then pass through the capillaries at the lungs and pick up oxygen to take out to the organs, tissues and cells again. This action from full movement of the diaphragm helps lighten the load on the cardiovascular system.

When we breathe fully and with intention, we are also improving our ability to manage stress and stress hormones. Intentional breathing helps us to restore balance between our sympathetic and parasympathetic branches of our autonomic nervous system. Some of the actions of the parasympathetic nervous system in the body include rest, digestion and assimilation of nutrients, and elimination of waste products. Time spent in this restful parasympathetic state on a regular basis allows the body to deal with minor repairs before they accumulate and become a very large problem. This parasympathetic state is also the body, mind and spirit's time to integrate new learned information and to grow and develop.

Some of the action of the sympathetic nervous system is often called the "fight or flight" response. The fight or flight response has gotten a bit of a bad reputation, however this reaction isn't a bad thing. It is perfectly designed if we need to do either of those activities, to fight or to flee. When our sympathetic nervous system is activated, our body chemistry changes so we can mobilize to ensure our survival. Problems can arise when we are perpetually in this fight or flight state. If you are fighting or running from a mountain lion, your body is in survival mode and isn't worried about performing repair or growth functions. It would be silly to devote energy to these activities if we're not sure if we'll be alive tomorrow. This means that our capacity to heal and grow is restricted as long as we live in sympathetic overdrive. That is why it is important to shift from sympathetic to parasympathetic mode, where the focus is on rest, repair, digestion/assimilation and elimination of waste products. Many of the chronic illnesses faced today are a result of living in sympathetic overdrive.

The fight or flight response is great - if you are actually going to fight or flee. It is perfectly designed to help you survive in the face of an immediate threat to your life and safety. It's not so great if you are going to continue to sit at your desk or in traffic, maintaining high levels of stress from day to day. The key to minimizing the damage that can result from a constant barrage of stress hormones is to move and breathe. In a true crisis situation where our survival is threatened, we would be intensely physically active and breathing fully as we were fighting off or fleeing from the potential threat. In our modern world, our stress response can trigger this dramatic cascade of stress hormones over work and school deadlines, family and relationship situations, traffic during our commute and other events that are more chronic in nature rather than an immediate threat to our survival.

There is another possible expression of the sympathetic nervous system activation besides fight or flight. It is the tendency to freeze. This is something we can observe in nature, particularly with prey animals. The animal senses a threat and freezes; hoping to go unnoticed if it remains still and quiet. I get to witness rabbits practice this freeze response while walking my dogs' daily. This response also shows up in us human animals. If we have been in a frightening or traumatic situation, we may freeze and hold our breath. I am very familiar with this particular expression, as it is one that I still catch myself doing now when under stress. Even when it is a positive stress, like learning something new, we may notice the tendency to hold the breath. Mindful breathing is a practice, not a quick fix. If you have been holding your breath as a response to stress for the majority of your life, that pattern isn't just going to disappear. The beautiful thing is that with practice you will notice the freeze response happening earlier and sooner, and you will spend less time in that state. With practice you may be able to anticipate situations that could prompt the freeze response and move immediately into mindful breathing to prevent that response from happening.

Once you are familiar with your mindful breathing practice, it is a wonderful thing to do while walking, dancing, practicing yoga, tai chi or qi gong, or any other physical activity you enjoy. If you are in a situation where you can't immediately move (like the traffic example mentioned earlier) this becomes a beautiful invitation to practice your intentional breathing in whatever situation you find yourself and flip the switch to a more healing and restorative state.

Regular time spent in a full, relaxed breathing pattern has been shown to lead to decreased pain perception, decreased blood levels of cortisol (the stress hormone), decreased stress perception, decreased levels of inflammatory markers in the blood (such as C reactive protein), and decreased hypertension (lowering high blood pressure). One way to prompt yourself to breathe more fully and deeply on a regular basis is to identify the breath deserts in your current life. Most people breathe in a very rapid and shallow fashion in a few common situations. Two of the biggest lifestyle offenders associated with this shallow, rapid breath pattern are driving and working at a computer. It is interesting to note that both activities also involve a sedentary, seated position. You may want to place something that reminds you of the breath in your car where you can see it when you first get inside. Then you can practice taking several deep breaths while sitting in the car before starting it up and rushing along your way. It can be helpful to post a sticker or a drawing that says BREATHE or reminds you of the breath near your desk as well. You may find it helpful to print out the Breath Check In Basics printable in the Bonus! section at the end of this book and hang it near your desk, in your bedroom, or in any areas where you would like to be reminded to breathe more fully. The benefit of using this printout is that in addition to providing a reminder, it also walks you through the steps of a mindful breathing practice.

Another way our mindful breathing practice can enhance our physical health is through helping us refine our understanding of our "edge," so we can prevent injury. When learning a new physical skill or challenging ourselves, we may experience intense physical sensations. Sometimes it can feel confusing and hard to tell if these sensations are due to muscular work or the very valuable warning signal of pain. When we breathe fully, it becomes easier to differentiate between the sensations of "work" and pain. Muscular effort can feel more manageable and less intense with full, intentional breathing. Pain that indicates that we need to change how we are moving or stop a particular activity will not undergo this same transformation when the breath is applied as a tool of discernment. Using our breath and awareness, we can begin to more successfully distinguish between "dang that's hard!" and "I better stop before I do any damage to myself".

Incredibly, mindful breathing can make a positive difference in our lives and our health by actually re-shaping our brains with regular practice. Mindful breathing enhances the quality of our lives by improving our ability to relate with kindness and compassion to ourselves and to others. It sharpens our ability to focus, learn, think, remember things and to regulate our emotions. Mindfulness increases our ability to empathize and to find perspective. These changes are due to measurable changes in specific areas of the brain that can occur in as little as eight weeks. Sara Lazar, a neuroscientist at Massachusetts General Hospital and Harvard Medical School, is someone devoted to studying these changes. Research done by Lazar and her team shows that the brains of people who engage in meditation and mindfulness practices, like Breathe Easy, show growth in the posterior cingulate gyrus, the left hippocampus, the temporo-parietal junction and the pons. An area of the brain called the amygdala (which is associated with stress, fear, and anxiety) shrunk over that same eight-week period. This decrease in size of the amygdala was unsurprisingly correlated with a reduction in stress levels of the study participants. The ability to change our brains in a measurable way seems like a pretty good reason to begin a daily mindful breathing practice now. Are you ready? Lets rock!

Chapter Sixteen

Final Integration and Putting it All Together

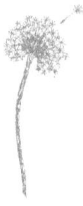

Now it's time for final integration and putting it all together. It is important to remember that the breath, like our posture, is constantly changing, moving, and adapting to best serve us in any particular situation. As we learn more about the breath, we can choose to vary the way we breathe to meet our needs depending on how we are feeling. A full, yet slightly faster breathing pattern can be more energizing if we are feeling tired and a long, smooth slower full breath pattern can be more calming and relaxing if we are feeling anxious or stressed. It is also highly beneficial to notice the breath as it shows up without changing it in any way to accurately assess how we are really feeling at any given time. Connecting with this free movement of the breath can give us a greater sense of the wisdom of the body as well as a fuller sense of our connection with all things. Lets play with integrating all of the elements that we have explored today, while we consider the details of how to create a daily practice.

BUILDING A DAILY PRACTICE

Moving forward, I encourage you to practice your *Breathe Easy* mindful breathing practice every day for best results. Use the Breath Check-In Basics printable (available in the Bonus! section) to help cue you through the important parts of checking in with your senses. You may also enjoy reading the daily practice notes that follow to review the parts of your body on which you would like to focus your awareness during your practice. Remember that this is an experiment and to just notice what is. You don't have to worry about doing things "right". If you keep showing up to your practice and watching your breath every day, the rest will take care of itself. There is no prescriptive amount of time for this practice, so feel free to tailor your practice to your day. You may want to begin with a shorter time interval like 3 minutes when first beginning this practice, or on days when you feel like your schedule is full. With time and experience, I encourage you to play with longer time periods, like 5, 10, 30, 45 or 60 minutes. You will figure out what works best for you each day.

When you begin practicing for longer periods of time, you may notice that your mind begins to wander to other thoughts that don't have anything to do with your breathing. This is okay and perfectly natural. It doesn't mean that you, or your practice, are a failure. It is a part of the practice. Minds think thoughts. Minds wander. When you catch your thoughts drifting to something other than your breath and how it is moving through your body, very gently redirect your awareness back to the breath. Use kindness and the type of patience you would use with a young child whom you love very much. We often talk to ourselves in ways that we would never speak to others and in ways that we would not tolerate from others. Develop a zero-tolerance policy for self-harm. This is a skill that takes time to grow and refine. Learning to show patience and kindness to yourself as you go through the sometimes-awkward process of learning a new skill like mindful breathing will have wonderful crossover and you will see that patience and kindness begin to show up in other areas of your life.

There will be some days when your mind is easily distractible and others when your focus is on point. Success in this sort of practice is not measured by which kind of day it is. That is a sneaky trap. Don't fall for it. Success in this type of practice is measured in your ability to show up for your practice day after day without expectation or getting attached to how you think your practice should look or feel.

The basics of developing a daily practice involve identifying what it takes for you personally to form a habit. This may mean practicing at the same time and in the same place every day... or it may not. That all will depend on who you are and what you need. There is that experiment piece showing up again. You may try many different approaches before settling into what feels like it works best for you. You may develop a set practice that works for years and then decide at some point that you want to change your approach. However you proceed, if you keep showing up for your practice you can't do it wrong.

You may want to find a quiet place to practice when you first begin and you may want to play with using music in the background. The advantage to not using music is that you can hear your breath more easily, while you may find that music may help you feel more relaxed at first if you are not accustomed to sitting in complete quiet. You may also enjoy using the audio Breathe Easy daily practice. The daily practice is about 15 minutes of detailed guided breath experience. This recording takes you through grounding into the sensory experience of your breath and connecting with the different areas of the body that are discussed in this book. When you want to focus on your breath and experience without having to guide yourself through your practice this can be a wonderful option.

A GUIDED BREATHE EASY PRACTICE

Find a comfortable place where you would like to practice your intentional breathing. You may choose to be seated, standing, lying down, or whatever other position feels the most comfortable to you right now.

Whatever position you choose, let yourself take a moment to connect with your foundation. Feel your body where it contacts the ground below and notice a sense of strength and stability that comes from that connection. As you feel ready, lengthen upward from that strong base. If you are sitting or standing, allow your spine and the crown of your head to lift toward the sky. If you are lying down, become aware of the long sense of spaciousness all along your spine from your tailbone to the top of your head. You may choose to let your eyes close at any point if that helps you to feel your breath.

Let your awareness be drawn to your breath. Feel the breath as it moves in and out through your nostrils. Allow yourself to observe your breath as it is right now without changing anything.

Become aware of the rate of your breath, whether it feels fast or slow.

Notice the depth of your breath, whether it feels shallow or deep.

Check in with the quality of your breath, noticing whether it is flowing smoothly or has rough edges.

Notice if there is any sound associated with your breath.

Are there are any emotions or feelings associated with this experience of your breath? Let yourself feel what is there without the need to get into any story around it.

Allow yourself to suspend any judgment about whether the way you are breathing is "good" or "bad" and let your self be fully present with what is. Notice where you feel your breath moving in your body. Gradually invite your breath to become more full and deep.

As you breathe in, allow your belly to gently soften and expand outward and downward. As you breathe out, gently draw your belly inward and upward to press out any stale air that may be lingering in the lower parts of your lungs. Allow the breath to begin to flow more deeply. With each inhale, draw your breath in and down so that it feels like your breath is flowing all the way down into the base of your pelvic bowl. As your belly gently expands outward, your pelvic floor expands downward. As you breathe out, gently draw your pelvic floor in and up, and draw your belly in and up as you exhale softly and completely.

As you take a breath in, visualize your breath traveling in and down through your nostrils, chest and abdomen, until it fills your pelvic bowl. As you breathe out, visualize the breath traveling up and out through your abdomen and chest, then exiting through your nostrils, as you feel a sense of energetic lift from the pelvic floor, upward through your body - traveling along the channel just forward of your spine. With each inhale, feel the breath flowing in and down - filling the body from the pelvic bowl, up though the abdomen, ribcage and chest. With each exhale, feel the softening - letting go of what you no longer need. Continue breathing in this slow smooth fashion.

Draw your awareness around to the sensations at the back of your body. With each inhale, feel the breath moving in and down along the channel just forward of your spine all the way until it reaches the tip of your tailbone. As you exhale, feel the breath trace that same path back up and out of the body as it leaves through the nostrils. With each inhale, feel a sense of expansion between your shoulder blades and a general broadening across the whole back body. With each exhale, feel a gentle sense of lift from your hip bones, upward through your waist along the spine.

Allow yourself to draw your awareness around to the sides of your body. With each breath in, notice a sense of expansion under your arms. With each breath out, feel the ribcage gently releasing. Inhale, feel your ribcage expanding out wide to the sides. Exhale, feel your ribcage soften.

Draw your awareness now to the breath as it flows freely on all sides of the body. With each inhale, feel the breath flowing in and down - filling the body from the pelvic bowl, up though the abdomen, ribcage and chest on all sides of the body. With each exhale, softening - letting go of what you no longer need. As you continue breathing in this slow smooth fashion, your body and mind become more and more deeply relaxed.

Begin to draw your awareness to the space between your ears and behind your eyes. With each breath in, feel an increasing sense of spaciousness and expansion within your head space. As you exhale, allow yourself to feel a gentle sense of lift, upward through the crown of your head - as if you are a whale softly spraying water up out of your spout. Inhale, feel the space between your ears broadening and your eyes softening. Exhale, feeling the crown of the head floating lightly upward. Continue with this smooth, full breath pattern at your own pace - feeling spaciousness on your inhale, and a sense of lift on your exhale.

Notice how you feel right now.

Check in with your physical body, becoming aware of any sensations calling out for your attention.

Notice your mental state and the quality and speed of your thoughts. Do not dive into any of the subjects of your thoughts at this point. Casually observe your thoughts as if from a distance and notice what's showing up for you now.

Check in with your subtle emotional body and again, take notice of what your feel.

Realize that there are no right or wrong answers here - only loving observation. Allow your awareness to fully return to your breath and where you feel it moving through your body.

As you breathe in, feel the breath drawing down deep into your body, feeling a sense of spaciousness and expansion on all sides of your body and within your head space. As you breathe out, feel a sense of lifting in and up as the muscles of your pelvic floor and belly begin the lift that starts the cascade of energy zipping upward - following the central channel just forward of your spine and outward through the crown of your head.

There is a dynamic pulse that flows through our breath and life of inhale/expansion, exhale/release. Allow yourself to feel this gentle pulse move through your entire body as you breathe. With each inhale, feel the physical body softly expanding in all directions. With each exhale, feel a sense of release and energetic lift. Continue feeling this pulse of life as you take five more breaths at your own pace. Feel free to close your eyes and focus on your breath and sensations if that is helpful to you. When you feel ready, you can gently blink your eyes open. In this way that you just experienced, the breath is a living and dynamic expression that flows through you.

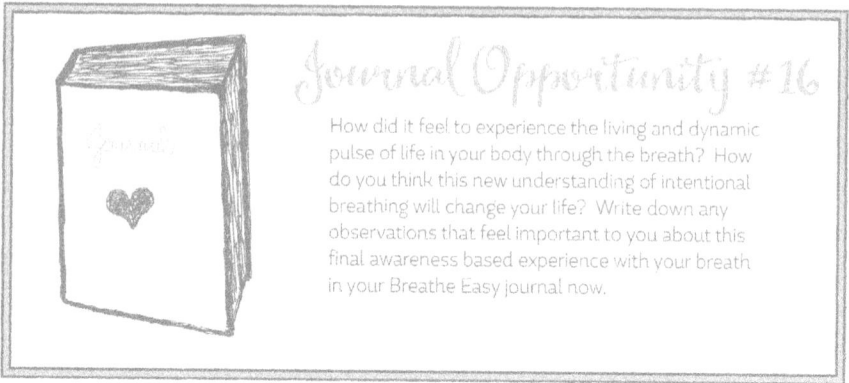

How did it feel to experience the living and dynamic pulse of life in your body through the breath? How do you think this new understanding of intentional breathing will change your life? Write down any observations that feel important to you about this final awareness based experience with your breath in your Breathe Easy journal now.

Take a moment to thank yourself for prioritizing your own loving self-care in the form of this breathing practice. Enjoy this sense of spaciousness you have created all day long by checking back in with your breath, noticing your thoughts and feeling the sensations in your body periodically throughout your day. With practice, you will begin to spend more and more time in this state of relaxation. It will become easier to connect with your breath and feel yourself maintaining a full breath pattern while you are going about your daily activities. The more time you spend in full breathing with awareness, the more you will begin to notice space between your thoughts and greater attention to the present moment. Allow yourself to engage your breathing practice while dancing, doing dishes, cuddling with pets or people, or any activity at all and be open to notice any transformation of that experience as you bring mindfulness and breathing into the mix.

I hope you have enjoyed learning about the breath and that you feel inspired to spend a few minutes checking in with your breath and breathing fully every day. Please use the printable graphic found in the Bonus! section as your daily breathing practice touchstone and revisit this e-book when you want to refine particular elements of your practice in greater detail.

I invite you to view each inhale is an opportunity to make a choice to nourish yourself, drawing in fresh and new vital energy. Each exhale is an invitation to soften your grip, soften your jaw, and soften your heart, as you let go of anything that no longer serves you.

Thank you so much for making your self-care a priority! It has been my honor and privilege to help you learn how to Breathe Easy and get Back In Body.

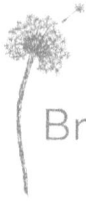

Breath Check-in
B A S I C S

▲ Connect with your foundation

LENGTHEN UP TALL ↟

Soft jaw, neck, & shoulders

notice your breath

DOES YOUR BREATH FEEL...

fast
-OR-
slow

shallow
-OR-
DEEP

smooth
-OR-
jagged

Does your breath carry any ♪Sounds♪

or ~emotions~ with it?

WHERE IS YOUR breath moving IN YOUR body?

♥ TAKE 10 FULL BREATHS ♥

Notice how you feel...
no right or wrong
just observation with love

Repeat
Often*

©2014 backinbody.com

Here is a gorgeous Breath Check-in Basics printable (designed by Gina Sekelsky of Lettergirl Studio) to help you connect with your breath at any time during the day. I encourage you to print several copies and hang them where you will see them. Hanging one by your desk, in your kitchen, or anywhere you do your movement or mindfulness practices will help remind you to breathe well and then guide you through the steps of connecting to the breath through sensory experience. Please feel free to print and share with people you love who might want to learn how to connect to their breathing too! There is a web address listed at the end of the Bonus section that will direct you where to go to access this free gift as well as the companion Breathe Easy journal.

Bonus!
Breathe Easy
Companion Journal

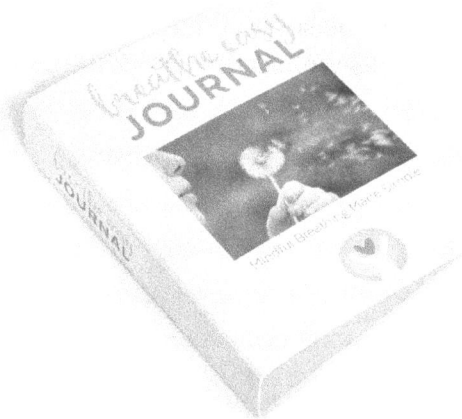

This is the companion _Breathe Easy_ journal that you can print out and assemble in any way you like to record your thoughts and feelings about your adventure in breathing! One suggestion for assembly is to get a three ring binder with a clear front pocket, print out the pdf and slide the cover in the front pocket, then three hole punch the inner pages and put them into the binder. You can use this journal as you follow along with the Journal Opportunity prompts in this book. In the future when you revisit the book, re-print the inner pages of the journal and record your experiences. If you do this, you will easily be able to see your understanding of your breath, and your relationship with your self, grow and change.

Please visit http://backinbody.com/breathe-easy-bonus-gifts/ to access both of your bonus gifts now!

I wish you continued love and luck on your breathing adventure!

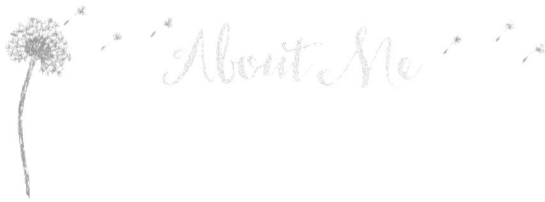

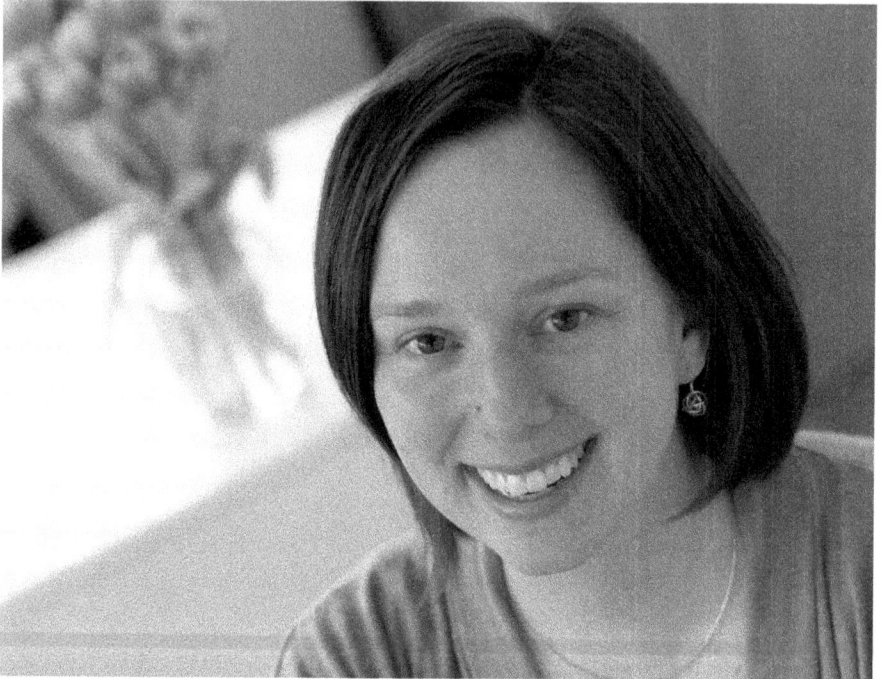

My name is Martha DeSante. I love breathing fully, eating well, bodywork, movement, creative pursuit, wildness and wilderness, living an embodied life and knowing it is all sacred.

My life purpose is to help people reconnect with their bodies and learn to inhabit them with love and joy. I help people heal from the wounds of denying themselves priority, pleasure and play. I have the amazing privilege of assisting people as they reclaim their power as the CEO of their health and wellness using the tools of the awesome chiropractic adjustment, muscle work (hands-on, Graston/Gua Sha), personally prescribed yoga, Pilates, and postural exercises, breath and awareness.

My goal in creating <u>Breathe Easy: mindful breathing made simple</u>, is to make the profound and amazing practice of mindful breathing as accessible as possible so that everyone can enjoy the benefits of better breathing.

Please visit my website at backinbody.com if you want to learn more about my educational and work experiences and the mission of my work with my company Back In Body.

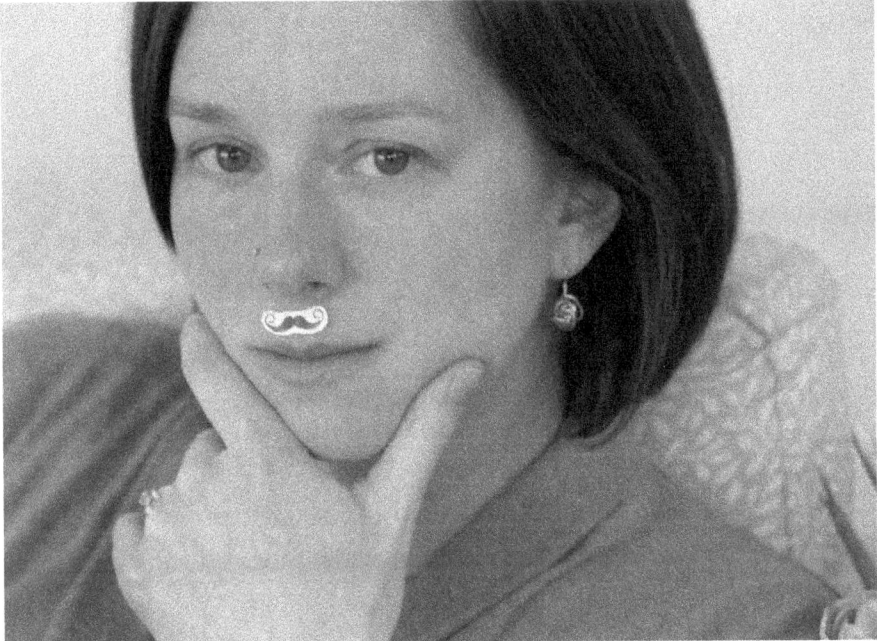

Mustache times are serious times.

Resources

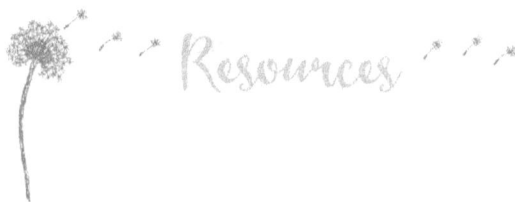

Here are some wonderful resources if you are interested in learning more about breathing, anatomy and how the body works in general!

HOW THE BODY IS PUT TOGETHER AND HOW IT WORKS

Calais-Germain, Blandine. Anatomy of Movement. Eastland Press: Seattle; WA, 1991.

Costanzo, Linda S. Physiology – Third Edition. Saunders Elsevier: Philadelphia; PA, 2006.

Coulter, H David. Anatomy of Hatha Yoga. Body and Breath Inc.: Honesdale; PA, 2001.

Dalley, Arthur F and Keith L Moore. Clinically Oriented Anatomy – Fifth Edition. Lippincott Williams & Wilkins: Baltimore; MD, 2006.

Hoehn, Katja and Elaine Nicpon Marieb. Human Anatomy and Physiology – Seventh Edition. Benjamin-Cummings: San Francisco; CA, 2006.

Netter, Frank H. Atlas of Human Anatomy. Saunders: Philadelphia; PA, 2006.

www.katysays.com and any resources by Katy Bowman

YOGA AND BREATHING

http://www.dailybandha.com/2013/11/sankalpa-visualization-and-yoga.html?m=1

Farhi, Donna. The Breathing Book. St. Martin's Press: New York; NY, 1996.

Iyengar, BKS. Light on Pranayama. Crossroad Publishing Company: New York; NY, 2013.

Rosen, Richard. The Yoga of Breath. Shambhala Publications: Boston, MA, 2002.

BREATHING THROUGH THE NOSE

Eddie Weitzberg and Jon O. N. Lundberg "Humming Greatly Increases Nasal Nitric Oxide", American Journal of Respiratory and Critical Care Medicine, Vol. 166, No. 2 (2002), pp. 144-145.

Elad, Wolf, Keck. 2008 Air-conditioning in the human nasal cavity. Respiratory Physioolgy and Neurobiology 163. 121-127

Settergren G, et al. (1998). Decreased pulmonary vascular resistance during nasal breathing: modulation by endogenous nitric oxide from the paranasal sinuses. Acta Physiol Scand. 1998 Jul;163(3):235-9.

Swift, Campbell, McKown. 1988 Oronasal obstruction, lung volumes, and arterial oxygenation. Lancet 1, 73-75.

Zinchuk VV. The involvement of nitric oxide in formation of hemoglobin oxygen-binding properties. Usp Fiziol Nauk, 2003 Apr-Jun;34(2):33-45.

BREATHING AND PELVIC FLOOR

Hodges, P.W., Sapsford, R. and Pengel, L.H.M. (2007), Postural and respiratory functions of the pelvic floor muscles. Neurourol. Urodyn., 26: 362–371. doi: 10.1002/nau.20232

Talasz H, et al. (2011). Phase-locked parallel movement of diaphragm and pelvic floor during breathing and coughing—a dynamic MRI investigation in healthy females. International Urogynecology Journal, 22 (1): 61-68

BREATHING AND POSTURE

Hodges, P. W., Heijnen, I. and Gandevia, S. C. (2001), Postural activity of the diaphragm is reduced in humans when respiratory demand increases. The Journal of Physiology, 537: 999–1008. doi: 10.1111/j.1469-7793.2001.00999.x

BREATHING DYSFUNCTION AND LOW BACK PAIN

Bradley H, Dr. and Esformes J. Breathing pattern disorders and functional movement. International Journal of Sports Physical Therapy. 2014;9(1):28-39.

Hagins M., and Lamberg EM, Individuals with low back pain breathe differently than healthy individuals during a lifting task. J Orthop Sports Phys Ther. 2011 Mar;41(3):141-8. doi: 10.2519/jospt.2011.3437. Epub 2011 Jan 4.

IMPROVING HEALTH CONDITIONS THROUGH BREATH PRACTICE

Asthma:
Thomas M, et al. Breathing retraining for dysfunctional breathing in asthma: a randomised controlled trial. Thorax 2003;58:110-115 doi:10.1136/thorax.58.2.110

Myasthenia Gravis:
Guilherme Augusto de Freitas Fregonezi, PT, MSc; Vanessa Regiane Resqueti, PT, MSc; Rosa Güell, MD, PhD; Jesus Pradas, MD, PhD; Pere Casan, MD, PhD. Effects of 8-Week, Interval-Based Inspiratory Muscle Training and Breathing Retraining in Patients With Generalized Myasthenia Gravis. Chest. 2005;128(3):1524-1530. doi:10.1378/chest.128.3.1524

BREATHING AND PAIN MANAGEMENT

Gard, T, Hölzel BK, Sack AT, et al. Pain Attenuation through Mindfulness is Associated with Decreased Cognitive Control and Increased Sensory Processing in the Brain. Cereb. Cortex (2012) 22 (11): 2692-2702. doi: 10.1093/cercor/bhr352.

BREATHING AND STRESS MANAGEMENT

Darviri C, Varvogli, L. (2011), Stress Management Techniques: evidence-based procedures that reduce stress and promote health. Health Science Journal. 2011; 5 (2).

Greenberg, Jerrold S. Comprehensive Stress Management – Seventh Edition. McGraw Hill: New York; NY, 2002.

Hölzel BK, Carmody J, Vangel M, et al. Mindfulness practice leads to increases in regional brain gray matter density. Psychiatry research. 2011;191(1):36-43. doi:10.1016/j.pscychresns.2010.08.006.

Hölzel BK, Carmody J, Karleyton CE, et al. Stress Reduction Correlates with Structural Changes in the Amygdala. Soc Cogn Affect Neurosci (2009) doi: 10.1093/scan/nsp034.2009.

Koene R. A. Van Dijk, Trey Hedden, Archana Venkataraman, et al. Intrinsic Functional Connectivity as a Tool For Human Connectomics: Theory, Properties and Optimization. Journal of Neurophysiology. 1 January 2010 Vol. 103 no. 1, 297-321 DOI: 10.1152/jn.00783.2009.

Lazar SW, Kerr CE, Wasserman RH, et al. Meditation experience is associated with increased cortical thickness. Neuroreport. 2005;16(17):1893-1897.

Lazar SW, Bush G, Gollub RL, et al. Functional Brain Mapping of the Relaxation Response and Meditation. Department of Psychiatry, Harvard Medical School, Massachusetts General Hospital-East, 5 March 2000.

Martarelli D, Cocchioni M, Scuri S, Pompei P. Diaphragmatic Breathing Reduces Exercise-Induced Oxidative Stress. Evidence-based Complementary and Alternative Medicine : eCAM. 2011;2011:932430. doi:10.1093/ecam/nep169.

BREATHING AND WEIGHT MANAGEMENT

Meerman R, Brown AJ. When somebody loses weight, where does the fat go? The BMJ, doi: 10.1136/bmj.g7257.

MINDFUL BREATHING AND INFLAMMATION REDUCTION

Creswell JD, Irwin MR, Burklund LJ, et al. Mindfulness-Based Stress Reduction Training Reduces Loneliness and Pro-Inflammatory Gene Expression in Older Adults: A Small Randomized Controlled Trial. Brain, behavior, and immunity. 2012;26(7):1095-1101. doi:10.1016/j.bbi.2012.07.006.

Sloan, R. P., et al. 2007. RR interval variability is inversely related to inflammatory markers: The CARDIA study. Mol Med 13 (3-4):178-84.